Anti Inflammat

100 Healthy Recipes

Kelly Bird

Recipe Junkies

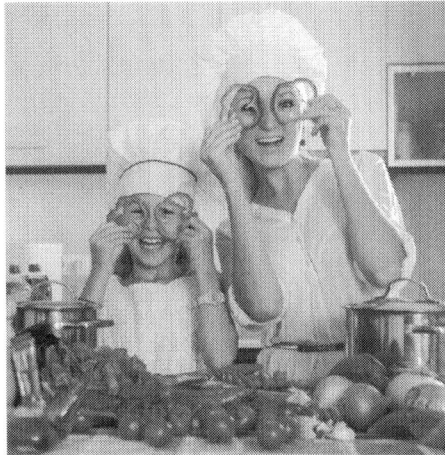

Poached Eggs and Curried Potatoes

Turkey Chili

Almond Chicken

Lemon-Almond Crusted Fish and Spinach

Chilled Habanero and Red Bell Pepper Soup

Rosemary Pecan Baked Tilapia

Stuffed Red Peppers Italian Style

Sweet Potato and Roasted Peppers Soup

Herbed Lemon Salmon and Zucchini

Spicy Black Bean Burgers

Curried Squash and Red Lentil Stew

Chicken and Kale Caesar Salad Wrap

Indian Spiced Carrot Ginger Soup

Pan Seared Salmon with Baby Arugula

Spinach, Goat Cheese and Bell Pepper Salad

Strawberry and Baby Spinach Salad

Lemon-Apricot Chicken and Cauli-Mash

Thai Rice Salad

American Casserole

Chop Suey with Light Salad

Arroz con Pollo

Asian Chicken Stir Fry

Avocado Chicken and Veggies

Baked Chicken and Broccoli Salad

Baked Cod with Beans

Fusilli Zucchini Bake

Baked Scallops

Barbecue Beef and Onions

Tomato Salad with Orzo and Barbecued Spiced Shrimp

Sausage and Bean Orzo

Barley and Beef Stir Fry

Cabbage and Beef Stir Fry

Red Wine Beef Stew

Beef Stroganoff

Chorizo and Black Bean Chili

Pork and Black Beans with Cauliflower and Broccoli

Braised Apple and Celery with Scallops

Broccoli Casserole

Broccoli Orzo

Broccoli and Ginger Chicken

Cajun Salmon

Chicken Cordon Bleu

Chicken Kali

Chicken Apple Pie

Chicken and Avocado Dip

Chicken Radicchio Salad

Shrimp and Chickpeas Mexicali

Chinese Orzo

Green Beans and Chorizo

Three Bean Salad and Chicken Marinara

Crab Bisque

Curried Eggplant

Lime and Dill Salmon

Cabbage Soup

Chicken Eggplant Parmigiana

Grill Bluefish

Eggplant Parmesan

Creamy Spicy Chicken Stew

Roasted Vegetables and Fusilli

Shrimp Fusilli with Asparagus and Roasted Tomatoes

Grilled Sole Filet and Leeks

Turkey and Mandarin Salad

Vegetable Beef Soup

Asian Style Halibut

Stir Fry Hot & Sour Pork with Cabbage

Shrimp, Yogurt and Apples Salad

Lentils and Italian Beef

Noodle-free Lasagna

Beef and Vegetable Stir Fry

Seafood Chowder

Meatloaf and Cheesy Veggies

Cashew Orange Chicken

Herbed Orange Chicken

Snow Peas and Oriental Turkey

Baked Overstuffed Portobello Mushroom

Papered Fish

Peking Shrimp

Poached Flounder

Vegetables with Pesto Sole

Tuscan Pork

Pork Fillet and Fennel

Pork Medallion with Blueberries and Pears

Apple Compote and Pork

Chicken Parmesan and Squash

Rosemary Chicken

Seared Salmon, Spinach and Balsamic Syrup

Salmon and Asian Fruit Salsa

Salsa Chicken

Braised Celery and Scallops

Seafood Pizza

Curried Eggplant and Salmon

Spanish Seafood Medley

Stuffed Peppers

Spaghetti with Cheesy Mushroom Sauce

Stuffed Zucchini

Sweet and Sour Shrimp

Teriyaki Halibut

Tofu Marinara

Baked Cabbage and Meatballs

Poached Eggs and Curried Potatoes

Serves: 4

Preparation Time: 40 minutes

Ingredients

Ginger (1 inch piece)

Olive oil (1 tablespoon)

Tomato sauce (15 oz.)

Cilantro

Russet potatoes (2 lbs.)

Garlic (2 cloves)

Curry powder (2 tablespoons)

Eggs (4, large)

Directions

1. Wash potatoes and then cut into cubes. Heat water in a large pot and add potatoes; cook for 6-10 minutes or until tender. Drain potatoes and put aside until needed (cover to keep warm).
2. Prepare sauce by removing peel from ginger and dice. Heat oil in a deep, large skillet and add garlic and ginger; sauté for 2 minutes or until garlic is fragrant. Put in curry and stir; cook for 1 minute.
3. Add tomato sauce and mix together then lower heat and allow sauce to cook until thoroughly heated. Add potatoes to mixture and use sauce to coat; add water in necessary.
4. Make 4 wells in potato mixture and break an egg into each. Cover pot and cook for 10 minutes or until eggs are set the way you prefer.
5. Serve topped with cilantro.

Nutritional Information

Calories 464 Carbs 50g Fat 13g Protein 13g

Turkey Chili

Serves: 8-10

Preparation Time: 4-6 hours

Ingredients

- Olive oil (1 tablespoon)
- Onion (1, chopped)
- Bell pepper (1 yellow, chopped)
- Canned tomatoes (30 oz., diced)
- Canned kidney beans (30 oz., drained and rinsed)
- Frozen corn (1 cup)
- Cumin (1 tablespoon)
- Ground turkey (1 lb., lean)
- Bell pepper (1 red, chopped)
- Tomato sauce (30 oz.)
- Canned black beans (30 oz., drained and rinsed)
- Jalapeno peppers (16 oz. jar, deli sliced, drained)
- Chili powder (2 tablespoons)

Directions

1. Heat oil in a skillet and cook turkey until golden; transfer turkey to slow cooker.
2. Add peppers, tomatoes, jalapenos, cumin, onion, tomato sauce, beans, chili powder and corn.
3. Set on low and cook for 6 hours or in high for 4 hours.
4. Serve as is or with desired toppings.

Nutritional Information

Calories 168

Carbs 27g

Fat 1g

Protein 13g

Almond Chicken

Serves: 2

Preparation Time: 30 minutes

Ingredients

Chicken breasts (6 oz., sliced)

Olive oil (3 teaspoons)

Red pepper (1, chopped)

Garlic (2 cloves, diced)

Salt

Almonds (4 teaspoons)

Broccoli florets (4 cups)

Green pepper (1, chopped)

Onion (1 ½ cups, chopped)

Cherry tomatoes (2 cups, sliced in halves)

Pepper

Directions

1. Place broccoli in a steamer or pot and cook for 5 minutes; put aside until necessary.
2. Heat oil in a skillet and sauté peppers, garlic, chicken and onion. Cook for 15 minutes or until thoroughly cooked.
3. Add broccoli and tomatoes to chicken; stir to combine and add pepper and salt to taste.
4. Serve topped with almonds

Nutritional Info

Calories 356 Carbs 40g Fat 11g

Protein 28g

Lemon-Almond Crusted Fish and Spinach

Serves: 4

Preparation Time: 50 minutes

Ingredients

Onions (1 ½ lbs.)

Vegetable stock (1 tablespoon, unsalted)

Balsamic vinegar (1/2 cup)

Almonds (1/2 cup, chopped)

Olive oil (2 teaspoons)

Codfish (1 lb.)

Water (1/4 cup)

Spinach (2 lbs.)

Olive oil (1 ½ teaspoons)

Orange juice (1/2 cup, freshly squeezed)

Lemon zest (from 1 lemon)

Dill (1 tablespoon, fresh)

Pepper

Dijon mustard (4 teaspoons)

Garlic (6 cloves, chopped)

Lemon juice (freshly squeezed)

Directions

1. Heat a pot of water and add onions; leave in water for 15 seconds then drain and add cold water to onions and drain again. Remove peels from onion and roots.
2. Heat stock and oil in a skillet and add onions; cook for 6 minutes until golden spots appear. Put in vinegar and orange juice and heat until it boils. Lower heat, stirring and scraping bits from pot; cook for 10 minutes until tender (use a knife

to test onion). Take onions from pot and put into a bowl and continue to boil for 3 minutes until mixture is syrupy. Pour sauce on top of onion and cover to keep warm.

3.   Set oven to 400°F and use cooking spray to coat a baking sheet. Mix together zest, dill, pepper, almonds and 2 teaspoons oil. Use 1 teaspoon mustard to spread onto each piece of fish then press into almond blend.

4.   Bake for 9 minutes while heating stock in a pot. Put in lemon juice, pepper and cook for 4 minutes. Add garlic, stir and cook for 2 minutes.

5.   Serve spinach along with fish.

Nutritional Info

Calories 371.5

Carbs 38g

Fat 12g

Protein 31g

Chilled Habanero and Red Bell Pepper Soup

Serves: 6

Preparation Time: 90 minutes

Ingredients

Bell peppers (4 red, medium)

Sweet onion (1/2 lb., chopped)

Habanero peppers (6. Seeds removed and diced)

Chicken broth (1 ¾ cups, low salt)

Tomatoes (2 lbs.)

Garlic (2 cloves, chopped)

Olive oil (1/4 cup, extra virgin)

Directions

1. Place bell peppers onto a greased baking sheet and broil for 10-15 minutes until blackened. Take from heat and place into a bowl; cover bowl with plastic wrap and put aside for 20 minutes. Remove the peel and slice peppers in half; discard seeds and stems.
2. Use a knife to score tomatoes with an X on the bottom of each then heat a pot of water and place tomatoes into pot for 20 seconds. Take from hot water and place into ice bath. Remove peel and chop; put aside till needed.
3. Heat 2 tablespoons oil and sauté habaneros, garlic and onion for 8 minutes or until golden and tender. Put in bell peppers, tomatoes and broth, cover and cook for 5 minutes or until bell peppers are soft.
4. Add oil to soup and puree in 2 or more batches or use an immersion blender to puree in pot then transfer soup to a metal bowl and chill in an ice bath, stirring frequently.
5. Serve.

Nutritional Info

Calories 211 Carbs 18g

Fat 15g

Protein 5g

Rosemary Pecan Baked Tilapia

Serves: 4

Preparation Time: 35 minutes

Ingredients

Panko breadcrumbs (1/3 cup)

Brown sugar (1/2 teaspoon)

Cayenne pepper

Egg white (1)

Raw pecans (1/3 cup, chopped)

Rosemary (2 teaspoons, chopped)

Olive oil (1 ½ teaspoons)

Tilapia (4 filets)

Directions

1. Set oven to 350°F.
2. Combine pecans, sugar, cayenne pepper and breadcrumbs together in a baking dish. Put in oil and mixture to coat.
3. Bake mixture for 8 minutes until golden.
4. Adjust oven temperature to 400°F. Use cooking spray to coat a baking dish and whisk egg white in a small dish. Coat filets one at a time with egg white and then with pecan mixture.
5. Place into greased baking dish and top with any leftover pecan mixture.
6. Bake for 10 minutes.
7. Serve.

Nutritional Info

Calories 206.5

Carbs 5.3g

Fat 10.1g

Protein 24.8g

Stuffed Red Peppers Italian Style

Serves: 4

Preparation Time: 35 minutes

Ingredients

Ground turkey/beef (1 lb., lean)

Spaghetti sauce (2 cups)

Garlic powder (1 teaspoon)

Spinach (1/2 cup, chopped)

Bell peppers (3 red)

Italian seasoning (1 teaspoon)

Vegan Parmesan (8 tablespoons)

Honey (1 teaspoon)

Directions

1. Set oven to 450° F.
2. Use foil to line a baking sheet and coat with cooking spray.
3. Wash bell peppers and remove stems. Slice peppers in half and take out seeds; place on prepared baking sheet.
4. Heat a skillet and cook turkey until slightly golden then add seasoning and sauce and mix together. Cook until turkey is done then add 2 tablespoons cheese and spinach; mix together and take from heat.
5. Spoon mixture into sliced peppers and top with leftover cheese.
6. Bake for 30 minutes until golden on top.
7. Serve warm.

Nutritional Info

Calories 170

Carbs 10g

Fat 8g

Protein 19g

Sweet Potato and Roasted Peppers Soup

Serves: 6

Preparation Time: 55 minutes

Ingredients

Olive oil (2 tablespoons)

Roasted red peppers (12 oz. jar, chopped with liquid)

Cumin (2 teaspoons)

Coriander (1 teaspoon)

Vegetable broth (4 cups)

Lemon juice (1 tablespoon)

Onions (2, chopped)

Green chilies (4 oz., diced)

Sweet potatoes (4 cups, peel removed and cubed)

Cilantro (2 tablespoons, chopped)

Vegan cream cheese (4 oz., cubed)

Directions

1. Heat oil in a soup pot and sauté onion for 3 minutes or until soft. Put in chilies, coriander, red peppers (without liquid) and cumin; cook for 2 minutes.
2. Add broth, liquid from peppers and sweet potatoes. Mix together and bring to a boil, lower flame and cover pot. Cook for 15 minutes until potatoes are cooked. Add lemon juice and cilantro; stir to combine and remove from heat.
3. Put cream cheese and half of soup in a processor and blend smoothly then add puree to remaining soup in pot and heat thoroughly,
4. Serve.

Nutritional Info

Calories 182 Carbs 40g Fat 2g

Protein 3g

Herbed Lemon Salmon and Zucchini

Serves: 4

Preparation Time: 35 minutes

Ingredients

Zucchini (4, chopped)

Black pepper

Olive oil (2 tablespoons)

For Salmon:

Lemon juice (2 tablespoons, freshly squeezed)

Garlic (2 cloves, diced)

Oregano (1/2 teaspoon, dried)

Rosemary (1/4 teaspoon, dried)

Salmon filets (4)

Brown sugar (2 tablespoons)

Dijon mustard (1 tablespoon)

Dill (1/2 teaspoon, dried)

Thyme (1/4 teaspoon)

Parsley (2 tablespoons, chopped)

Directions

1. Set oven to 400F and use cooking spray to coat a baking sheet.
2. Combine lemon juice, dill, thyme, sugar, mustard, rosemary and oregano together in a small bowl and put aside till needed.
3. Put zucchini onto baking sheet and use oil to drizzle all over. Coat one side of fish with herb blend and place onto baking sheet.
4. Bake for 16-18 minutes or until fish is flaky.
5. Serve topped with parsley.

Nutritional Info

Calories 220 Carbs 11g Fat 14g

Protein 23g

Spicy Black Bean Burgers

Serves: 6

Preparation Time: 60 minutes

Ingredients

Quinoa (1/2 cup)

Sweet potato (1)

Garlic (2 cloves, diced)

Jalapeno (1/2, seed removed and chopped)

Cajun seasoning (2 teaspoons)

Coconut oil

Sprouts

Black beans (15 oz., drained and rinsed)

Red onion (1/2 cup, chopped)

Cilantro (1/2 cup, chopped)

Cumin (1 teaspoon)

Oat flour (1/4 cup)

Hamburger buns (6, whole grain)

For Avocado Crema:

Sour cream (1/4 cup, low fat)

Lime juice (1 teaspoon)

Avocado (1/2, chopped)

Cilantro (2 tablespoons)

Hot sauce

Directions

1. Prepare quinoa as directed on package and put aside until needed.
2. Use a fork to pierce potato and put into microwave for 4 minutes or until thoroughly cooked. Remove peel and place into a food processor along with beans, cilantro, cumin, onion, Cajun seasoning and garlic. Combine all ingredients and out mixture into a bowl.
3. Add quinoa to bean mixture and combine (add more Cajun seasoning if so desired); add oat flour and combine. Divide mixture into 6 equal parts and use hands to shape. Put onto baking sheet and chill for 30 minutes.
4. Make crema by combining all ingredients in a processor until smooth; put into refrigerator until needed.
5. Heat coconut oil in a skillet and cook patties for 4 minutes on both sides.
6. Assembly burgers by placing patties on buns and topping with sprouts and crema.

Nutritional Info (without bun)

Calories 206

Carbs 33.9g

Fat 6g

Protein 7.9g

Curried Squash and Red Lentil Stew

Serves: 4

Preparation Time: 30 minutes

Ingredients

Olive oil (1 teaspoon)

Garlic (3 cloves, diced)

Broth (4 cups, low salt)

Butternut squash (3 cups, cooked)

Ginger (grated)

Sweet onion (1, chopped)

Curry powder (1 tablespoon)

Red lentils (1 cup)

Spinach (1 cup)

Herb seasoning (1/2 teaspoon)

Directions

1. Heat oil in a soup pot and sauté onion for 3 minutes or until soft. Put in chilies, coriander, red peppers (without liquid) and cumin; cook for 2 minutes.
2. Add broth, liquid from peppers and sweet potatoes. Mix together and bring to a boil, lower flame and cover pot. Cook for 15 minutes until potatoes are cooked. Add lemon juice and cilantro; stir to combine and remove from heat.
3. Put cream cheese and half of soup in a processor and blend smoothly then add puree to remaining soup in pot and heat thoroughly,
4. Serve.

Nutritional Info

Calories 145 Carbs 25g

Fat 2g

Protein 9g

Chicken and Kale Caesar Salad Wrap

Serves: 2

Preparation Time: 10 minutes

Ingredients

Grilled chicken (8 oz., sliced thin)

Cherry tomatoes (1 cup, cut into quarters)

Coddled egg (1/2)

Dijon mustard (1/2 teaspoon)

Lemon juice (1/8 cup, freshly squeezed)

Flat bread/Tortillas (2)

Curly kale (6 cups, chopped)

Vegan Parmesan (3/4 cup, shredded)

Garlic (1 clove, diced)

Honey (1 teaspoon)

Olive oil (1/8 cup)

Directions

1. Put coddled egg, mustard, lemon juice, olive oil and garlic together in a bowl; whisk together until thoroughly combined.
2. Add tomatoes, chicken and kale to mixture and coat then add ¼ cup of cheese.
3. Divide salad in 2 and spoon onto tortillas/flatbread and top with 1/4cup cheese each.
4. Roll wraps and cut into half.
5. Serve.

Nutritional Info

Calories 323 Carbs 21g

Fat 11g

Protein 34g

Indian Spiced Carrot Ginger Soup

Serves: 6-8

Preparation Time: 40 minutes

Ingredients

Coriander seeds (1 teaspoon)

Peanut oil (3 tablespoons)

Ginger (1 tablespoon, peeled and diced)

Carrots (1 ½ lbs., sliced thin into rounds)

Chicken broth (6 cups, low salt)

Mustard seeds (1/2 teaspoon, yellow)

Curry powder (1/2 teaspoon)

Onion (2 cups, chopped)

Lime zest (1 ½ teaspoons)

Lime juice (2 teaspoons, freshly squeezed)

Directions

1. Grind mustard seeds and coriander together finely.
2. Heat oil in a large soup pot and add curry powder along with ground mixture then add ginger and cook for 1 minute.
3. Add zest, onion and carrots; cook for 3 minutes until onions are soft then add broth and heat until mixture boils.
4. Lower heat and cook for 30 minutes until carrots are cooked. Remove from heat and allow to cool.
5. Puree in batches or use an immersion blender to puree. Reheat, adding more liquid if necessary along with lime juice.
6. Serve.

Nutritional Info

Calories 163 Carbs 19g Fat 8g

Protein 6g

Pan Seared Salmon with Baby Arugula

Serves: 2

Preparation Time: 25 minutes

Ingredients

Salmon (2 center cut filets)

Olive oil (1 ½ tablespoons)

Black pepper

Lemon juice (1 ½ tablespoons)

All purpose seasoning (1/8 teaspoon)

For salad:

Cherry tomatoes (2/3 cup, cut in half)

Black pepper

Wine vinegar (1 tablespoon)

Baby arugula (3 cups)

Red onion (1/4 cup, sliced)

Olive oil (1 tablespoon, extra virgin)

Directions

1. Season fish with all purpose, oil and lemon juice; marinate for 15 minutes.
2. Heat skillet and place the salmon onto the skin side into the pot and cook for 3 minutes. Use a spatula to lightly lift fish to avoid sticking.
3. Lower heat and cover pan; cook for 4 minutes until skin is crispy.
4. Combine onion, tomatoes and arugula in a bowl then drizzle with vinegar and oil.
5. Serve salad with fish.

Nutritional Info

Calories 390 Carbs 4g Fat 23g

Protein 40g

Spinach, Goat Cheese and Bell Pepper Salad

Serves: 4

Preparation Time: 10 minutes

Ingredients

Olive oil (2 tablespoons, extra-virgin)

Oregano (1 tablespoon, chopped)

Red peppers (1 ½ large, diced)

Goat cheese (3/4 cup, soft, crumbled)

Lemon juice (2 tablespoon, freshly squeezed)

Spinach leaves (4 cup, chopped)

Red onion (1/3 cup, chopped)

Celery (1 ½ cups, chopped)

Directions

1. Put oregano, lemon juice and oil in a bowl and whisk together.
2. Add remaining ingredients to dressing and toss.
3. Serve. May be chilled before serving.

Nutritional Info

Calories 155

Carbs 0g

Fat 11g

Protein 0g

Strawberry and Baby Spinach Salad

Serves: 1

Preparation Time: 15 minutes

Ingredients

For salad:

Baby spinach (3 cups, remove stems)

Red onion (1/4, sliced thin)

Garbanzo beans (1/4 cup, drained and rinsed)

Portobello mushroom (1 cup, chopped)

Strawberries (10, sliced)

Chicken breasts (1/2 cup, cooked without skin)

For dressing:

Shallot (1 teaspoon, diced)

Orange zest (1/4 teaspoon, grated)

Black pepper (1/8 teaspoon)

Olive oil (1 ½ teaspoons)

Champagne vinegar (1 tablespoon)

Orange juice (1 tablespoon, freshly squeezed)

Directions

1. Rinse spinach and set aside in a colander to drain dry.
2. Put spinach into a bowl with all remaining ingredients for salad.
3. Heat oil in a skillet and add shallots, orange zest, pepper and vinegar; cook for 3 minutes.
4. Add orange juice to dressing and whisk to combine.
5. Pour dressing on top of salad, toss and serve.

Nutritional Info

Calories 353 Carbs 34g Fat 11g

Protein 32g

Lemon-Apricot Chicken and Cauli-Mash

Serves: 4

Preparation Time: 40 minutes

Ingredients

Baby spinach (8 cups)

Strawberries (1 cup, sliced)

Red onion (1 cup, sliced)

Curry powder (1 teaspoon)

Black pepper (1/4 teaspoon)

Apricot preserves (1/3 cup, sugar-free)

Water (2 tablespoons)

Apples (2)

Mushrooms (8 oz., sliced)

Blueberries (1/2 cup)

Balsamic dressing (1/2 cup, light)

Chicken breast (14 oz., without skin or bone)

Lemon juice (2 tablespoons, freshly squeezed)

Lemon zest (2 teaspoons, grated)

For 'Mashed Potatoes':

Frozen cauliflower (16 oz.)

Greek yogurt (3 ½ tablespoons, no fat)

Black pepper

Chicken broth (2 tablespoons, unsalted)

Olive oil (1 tablespoon, extra-virgin)

Directions

1. Prepare cauli-mash by putting cauliflower and broth into a microwavable dish and microwave for 12 minutes. Do not overcook, should be slightly crunchy.
2. Transfer cooked cauliflower to a food processor along with yogurt and black pepper. Pulse mixture until cauliflower has a mashed potato consistency. Drizzle with oil and put aside till needed.
3. Combine mushrooms, red onion, spinach and strawberries in a bowl; put aside in fridge until needed.
4. Season chicken with curry and black pepper. Use cooking spray to coat a skillet and cook chicken for 5 minutes on both sides or until thoroughly cooked.
5. Take chicken from pot and add lemon juice, water and preserves; mix together until smooth.
6. Serve cauli-mash with chicken, drizzle with sauce on chicken and add salad with dressing.

Nutritional Info

Calories 269

Carbs 17g

Fat 2g

Protein 39g

Thai Rice Salad

Serves: 1

Preparation Time: 20 minutes

Ingredients

For salad:

Orzo pasta (1/3 cup)

Scallions (2, chopped)

Baby bok choy (1 cup, chopped)

Basil (2 tablespoons, chopped)

Asparagus (1/3 lb., chopped)

Carrot (1/4 cup, grated)

Cilantro (2 tablespoons, chopped)

For dressing:

Olive oil (1 ½ teaspoons, extra-virgin)

Thai fish sauce (1 teaspoon)

Ginger (1 teaspoon, grated)

Lime juice (1 ½ teaspoons, freshly squeezed)

Sweet chili sauce (1 tablespoon)

Cayenne pepper

Directions

1. Prepare pasta as directed on package.
2. Add asparagus to pasta in the final 2 minutes of cooking, drain and run under cold water. Drain again and put aside to cool.
3. Add cooked pasta and asparagus to a bowl along with scallions, bok choy, carrot, basil and cilantro; toss to combine.
4. Put all ingredients for dressing into another bowl and drizzle over rice salad.

5. Serve.

Nutritional Info

Calories 318

Carbs 37g

Fat 10g

Protein 20g

American Casserole

Serves: 6

Preparation Time: 50 minutes

Ingredients

Fusilli (4 ½ cups, organic)

Ground turkey breast (5 oz.)

Bell pepper (1 cup, chopped)

Green beans (16 oz.)

Water (1 cup)

Basil (1 teaspoon, dried)

Vegan mozzarella (3/4 cup)

Olive oil (1 tablespoon)

Roma tomatoes (4, chopped)

Onion (1 ½ cups, chopped)

Tomato sauce (26 oz.)

Italian seasoning (1 teaspoon)

Black pepper

Directions

1. Set oven to 350F. Use cooking spray to coat casserole dish and put aside until needed.
2. Heat oil in a skillet and sauté onion, bell pepper and tomatoes for 1 minute then add turkey and cook for 5 minutes until golden.
3. Add tomato sauce, fusilli, black pepper, green beans, water and spices. Stir to combine and cook for 15 minutes or until fusilli is thoroughly cooked.
4. Put into greased casserole dish, cover with foil and bake for 25 minutes.
5. Take from oven and top with cheese and bake for an additional 10 minutes without cover.
6. Top with a little oil and serve.

Nutritional Info

Calories 358 Carbs 40g Fat 9g Protein 28g

Chop Suey with Light Salad

Serves: 1

Preparation Time: 20 minutes

Ingredients

Fusilli (3/4 cups, organic)

Celery (1/2 stalk, chopped)

Garlic (1 clove, diced)

Ground turkey (1.5 oz., lean)

Red pepper flakes (1/4 teaspoon)

Black pepper

Water (1 tablespoon)

Olive oil (1 teaspoon, extra-virgin)

Onion (1/2, chopped)

Bell pepper (1/2, chopped)

Canned tomatoes (7 oz., diced)

Basil (1/4 teaspoon, chopped)

Lemon juice (1 tablespoon, freshly squeezed)

For Salad:

Lettuce (1/2 cup)

Cucumber (1/4 cup)

Olive oil (1/2 teaspoon)

Bell pepper (1/4, sliced)

Directions

1.   Cook fusilli for 4 minutes, drain and put aside.

2. Heat oil in a skillet and sauté onion and celery for 3 minutes then add bell pepper and garlic; take from pot and put aside.
3. Use cooking spray to coat pot and cook turkey for 5 minutes or until thoroughly golden.
4. Add fusilli and cooked vegetables to pot along with crushed pepper and canned tomatoes; mix together, cover and cook for 8 minutes.
5. Top with basil and serve. Combine ingredients for salad and serve alongside chop suey.

Nutritional Info

Calories 365

Carbs 39g

Fat 11g

Protein 28g

Arroz con Pollo

Serves: 1

Preparation Time: 15 minutes

Ingredients

Olive oil (1 ½ teaspoons)

Garlic (1/2 clove, diced)

Water (1/4 cup)

Bay leaves (1/2 teaspoon)

Green beans (1/2 cup, chopped)

Orzo (1/3 cup)

Onion (1/4, diced)

Tomato sauce (1/4 cup)

Vegetable broth (4 oz.)

Oregano (1/2 teaspoon, dried)

Chicken breast (1/4 cup)

Black pepper

Directions

1. Prepare orzo as directed on package; drain and put aside till needed.
2. Heat ½ teaspoon oil in a skillet and cook garlic and onion for 3 minutes.
3. Add water, bay leaves, oregano, tomato sauce and broth; stir to combine and add black pepper to taste.
4. Add green beans, mix together and cook for 8 minutes then add chicken and orzo; cook for 2 minutes.
5. Top with oil and serve.

Nutritional Info

Calories 345 Carbs 35g Fat 12g

Protein 26g

Asian Chicken Stir Fry

Serves: 2

Preparation Time: 30 minutes

Ingredients

Olive oil (2 teaspoons)

Garlic (2 cloves, crushed)

Mushrooms (8 oz., sliced)

Snow peas (1 cup)

Soy sauce (2 teaspoons, low salt)

Sesame oil (1 teaspoon)

Broccoli (3 cups, chopped)

Chicken breast (7 oz., cubed)

Water chestnuts (3/4 cup, sliced)

Red bell pepper (1, sliced)

Scallions (1/2 cup, chopped)

Mandarin (1/2 cup)

Directions

1. Steam broccoli for 4 minutes then run under water and drain.
2. Heat oil in a skillet and add garlic and chicken; cook for 10 minutes.
3. Add mushrooms, snow peas, soy sauce, chestnuts, pepper and scallions.
4. Cook for 15 minutes, stirring occasionally then add sesame oil and mandarin.
5. Serve.

Nutritional Info

Calories 359 Carbs 39g

Fat 11g

Protein 31g

Avocado Chicken and Veggies

Serves: 1

Preparation Time: 45 minutes

Ingredients

Avocado (1 tablespoon)

Chicken breast (3 oz., skinless)

Zucchini (1 cup, sliced)

Onions (1/2 cup, chopped)

Vegetable stock (1/4 cup, no salt)

Basil (2 teaspoons, dried)

Cream cheese (1 tablespoon, low fat)

Black pepper

Herb seasoning

Mushrooms (1 cup, sliced)

Green beans (3/4 cup)

Canned tomatoes (14.5 oz., diced with liquid)

Olive oil (1 teaspoon, extra-virgin)

Directions

1. Set oven to 350F.
2. Combine cream cheese and avocado using a fork to mash.
3. Use a knife to make a pocket in the chicken breast and stuff with avocado mixture; use toothpicks to seal.
4. Use cooking spray to coat a baking sheet and season chicken with black pepper and herb seasoning.
5. Bake for 25 minutes.
6. Coat skillet with cooking spray and add vegetables (excluding tomatoes) and stock to pot. Cook for 5 minutes or until tender then add tomatoes and heat thoroughly.

7. Serve chicken with vegetables; drizzle oil over vegetables.

Nutritional Info

Calories 351

Carbs 40g

Fat 12g

Protein 29g

Baked Chicken and Broccoli Salad

Serves: 2

Preparation Time: 45 minutes

Ingredients

Chicken breast (4 oz., skinless and boneless)

Broccoli (5 cups, chopped)

Carrots (1/3 cup, shredded)

Greek yogurt (1/2 cup, no fat)

Lemon juice (1 tablespoon, freshly squeezed)

Black pepper

Herb seasoning

Turkey bacon (4 slices)

Canned water chestnuts (3 oz., chopped)

Sesame seeds (1 tablespoon)

Mayonnaise (2 teaspoons, light)

Garlic powder (1/2 teaspoon)

Canned peaches (1 ½ cups, drained)

Directions

1. Set oven to 350F.
2. Season chicken with herb seasoning, coat baking tray with cooking spray and place chicken onto try; bake for 35 minutes.
3. Heat skillet and cook bacon until crisp. Put aside on paper towels to remove excess oil.
4. Combine broccoli, carrots, sesame seeds and water chestnuts in a bowl. Mix together mayonnaise, garlic powder, pepper, yogurt and lemon juice and add to salad; toss to combine.
5. Add peaches and chicken and top with bacon.
6. Serve.

Nutritional Info

Calories 358 Carbs 38g Fat 12g Protein 31g

Baked Cod with Beans

Serves: 1

Preparation Time: 30 minutes

Ingredients

Olive oil (2 teaspoons)

Cod (4 oz.)

Green beans (2 cups)

Blueberries (1/2 cup)

Old-fashioned oats (1 tablespoon)

Tomato (2 slices)

Directions

1. Set oven to 400°F.
2. Combine oats and half of oil in a bowl and use mixture to coat fish.
3. Coat baking tray with cooking spray and place fish onto tray and top with the tomato slices and bake for 15 minutes.
4. Steam green beans and serve with fish and blueberries.

Nutritional Info

Calories 350

Carbs 39g

Fat 11g

Protein 27g

Fusilli Zucchini Bake

Serves: 1

Preparation Time: 30 minutes

Ingredients

Fusilli pasta (2/3 cup, organic)

Zucchini (1/2 cup, cubed)

Canned tomatoes (7 oz., diced)

Water (2 tablespoons)

Canadian bacon (1 slice, chopped)

Vegan mozzarella cheese (2 tablespoons, shredded)

Olive oil (1 teaspoon)

Green beans (1/2 cup, sliced)

Tomato sauce (1/2 cup)

Italian seasoning (1/4 teaspoon)

Black pepper

Vegan Parmesan (1 teaspoon, grated)

Directions

1. Set oven to 375F.
2. Heat oil in a skillet and add green beans and zucchini. Cook for 5 minutes with cover, stirring occasionally to avoid burning.
3. Add tomatoes, water, bacon, black pepper, tomato sauce and Italian seasoning; stir to combine and cook for 4 minutes.
4. Prepare pasta as directed on package, drain and add to cooked vegetables.
5. Use cooking spray to coat baking dish and add mixture to dish. Top with cheeses and bake with cover for 10 minutes.
6. Remove cover and bake for 10 minutes more.
7. Serve warm.

Nutritional Info

Calories 352 Carbs 40g Fat 11g

Protein 25g

Baked Scallops

Serves: 1

Preparation Time: 30 minutes

Ingredients

Bay scallops (3 oz.)

Oats (1 tablespoon, old-fashioned)

Olive oil (1 ½ teaspoons, extra-virgin)

Lemon pepper

Garbanzo beans (1/4 cup, low salt)

Cucumber (1 cup)

White wine (3 tablespoons)

Cheddar cheese (1/2 oz., low fat, shredded)

Lemon juice (3 tablespoons, freshly squeezed)

Romaine lettuce (3 cups, chopped)

Tomato (1)

Directions

1. Put scallops into a container and cover with white wine; cover container and put into refrigerator overnight.
2. Set oven to 350F.
3. Remove scallops from wine and top with oats and cheese.
4. Place onto a baking tray and bake for 10 minutes.
5. Combine lemon pepper, lemon juice and oil in a small bowl.
6. Mix together garbanzo beans, cucumber, lettuce and tomato.
7. Serve salad topped with lemon dressing and baked scallops.

Nutritional Info

Calories 358 Carbs 34g Fat 11g

Protein 27g

Barbecue Beef and Onions

Serves: 1

Preparation Time: 45 minutes

Ingredients

Olive oil (1 ½ teaspoons)

Tomato puree (1/2 cup)

Cider vinegar (1/3 teaspoon)

Cumin (1/8 teaspoon)

Onion (1 cup, sliced)

Mushrooms (1 cup)

White wine vinegar (2 teaspoons)

Beef (3 oz., eye of round)

Worcestershire sauce (1 teaspoon)

Chili powder (1/3 teaspoon)

Oregano (1/8 teaspoon)

Garlic (1 clove, diced)

Vegetable stock (2 teaspoons, no salt)

Snow peas (1 cup)

Directions

1. Heat ½ teaspoon oil in a skillet and cook beef for 10 minutes.
2. Add Worcestershire sauce, chili powder, oregano, tomato puree, cider vinegar and cumin; cook for 5 minutes with pot covered.
3. Heat remaining oil in another skillet and sauté garlic and onion for 5 minutes until tender.
4. Add sautéed mixture to beef along with vinegar, stock and mushrooms; cover pot and cook for 8 minutes.
5. Put in snow peas and cook for 5 minutes; mix together to combine.
6. Serve.

Nutritional Info

Calories 368 Carbs 36g Fat 12g Protein 32g

Tomato Salad with Orzo and Barbecued Spiced Shrimp

Serves: 2

Preparation Time: 40 minutes

Ingredients

Orzo pasta (2/3 cup)

Olive oil (1 tablespoon)

Black pepper

Chile powder (1/2 teaspoon, ancho)

Cumin (1/4 teaspoon)

Cayenne pepper

Lime juice (3 tablespoons, freshly squeezed)

Red onion (1/2, sliced)

Basil leaves (2 tablespoons)

Smoked paprika (1 teaspoon)

Agave nectar (1 teaspoon)

Coriander (1/4 teaspoon)

Jumbo shrimp (3 oz., deveined and without shell)

Lettuce (8 leaves)

Tomatoes (2, sliced)

Directions

1. Put oil and basil into a processor or blender and pulse until smooth. Add black pepper and lime juice, mx together and put aside until needed.
2. Heat grill.
3. Combine chili powder, cumin, cayenne pepper, paprika, sugar and coriander in a small bowl.

4. Coat shrimp with cooking spray and spice blend and put aside; prepare orzo as directed on package, run under cold water and drain.
5. Pour lime juice over orzo.
6. Grill shrimp for 4 minutes until slightly charred.
7. Place lettuce on a place and top with orzo, onion and tomato and drizzle with basil blend.
8. Add shrimp and serve.

Nutritional Info

Calories 345

Carbs 35g

Fat 11g

Protein 26g

Sausage and Bean Orzo

Serves: 2

Preparation Time: 20 minutes

Ingredients

Tomatoes (1/2 lb., cooked)

Chicken sausage (2 cups, sliced)

Onion (1/2, chopped)

Cannellini beans (1/2 cup, canned)

Water (4 cups)

Olive oil (2 teaspoons)

Orzo (2/3 cup)

Garlic (1 clove, diced)

Cilantro (2 tablespoons, chopped)

Black pepper

Directions

1. Put the cooked tomato, black pepper and water into a blender/processor and blend together; put aside until needed.
2. Heat oil in a saucepan and cook sausage until browned; take from pot and put aside.
3. Add onion and orzo to the same pot and cook for 3 minutes until golden then add garlic, stir and cook for an additional minute.
4. Add puree to pot, cover and cook for 15 minutes until thoroughly cooked.
5. Put in sausage and beans and cook for an additional 5 minutes.
6. Serve topped with cilantro.

Nutritional Info

Calories 374 Carbs 39g Fat 12g

Protein 27g

Barley and Beef Stir Fry

Serves: 2

Preparation Time: 20 minutes

Ingredients

Barley (1/4 cup, pearled)

Olive oil (2 teaspoons)

Onions (3/4 cup, chopped)

Green beans (2 cups)

Soy sauce (1/2 teaspoon, low salt)

Tomato (1, sliced)

Ground beef (7 oz., lean)

Mushrooms (1 cup)

Vegetable broth (1/4 cup, no salt)

Directions

1. Prepare barley as directed on package, drain and put aside until needed.
2. Heat oil in skillet and add beef to pot; cook until meat is golden then add green beans, mushrooms and onion. Mix together and cook until beans are tender.
3. Add soy sauce and broth to cooked barley and mix together then add to vegetable and meat.
4. Serve with tomato.

Nutritional Info

Calories 355

Carbs 38g

Fat 10g

Protein 28g

Cabbage and Beef Stir Fry

Serves: 4

Preparation Time: 40 minutes

Ingredients

Peanut butter (2 ½ tablespoons, low fat)

Soy sauce (3 tablespoons, low salt)

Rice vinegar (1 tablespoon)

Garlic (3 cloves, diced)

Cabbage (1 head, sliced thin)

Beef stock (4 tablespoons)

Peanuts (4 teaspoons, chopped)

Orange juice (1/3 up, freshly squeezed)

Water (4 tablespoons)

Olive oil (1 teaspoon)

Sirloin steak (14 oz., sliced thin)

Bell peppers (2, red, sliced thin)

Carrots (4, grated)

Mandarin (1 cup)

Directions

1. Whisk orange juice, I tablespoon stock, vinegar and peanut butter together in a bowl; put aside until needed.
2. Heat oil in a skillet and sauté garlic for 1 minute until fragrant.
3. Put steak into pot and cook for 4 minutes then add a little stock. Take from pot and place aside in a bowl.
4. Lower heat and add leftover stock and cabbage, cook for 5minutes until it wilts then put in carrots and a little water, stir and cook for 3 minutes.
5. Add steak to pot again along with any liquid and peanut sauce; toss to combine.

6. Top with peanuts and serve along with mandarin.

Nutritional Info

Calories 364

Carbs 35g

Fat 12g

Protein 28g

Red Wine Beef Stew

Serves: 4

Preparation Time: 1 hour 20 minutes

Ingredients

Olive oil (1 ½ teaspoons)

Onion (1 ½ cups, diced)

Parsley (1/4 cup, chopped)

Bay leaf (1)

Nutmeg (1/2 teaspoon)

Canned tomatoes (14 oz., diced with liquid)

Black pepper

Beef (6 oz., boneless, cubed)

Carrots (2, chopped)

Garlic (2 cloves, chopped)

Thyme (1/2 teaspoon)

Red Wine (1/2 cup)

Beef broth (3/4 cup, no salt)

Bell peppers (2, sliced)

Directions

1. Set oven to 350F.
2. Heat oil in a skillet and cook meat until browned then take from pot and put aside.
3. Add carrots and onion to pot and cook for 3 minutes until tender; add garlic and parsley and cook for an additional 3 minutes.
4. Add semi-cooked meat to vegetables in pot and mix together.
5. Add nutmeg, thyme, bay leaf and wine; cook for 4 minutes, stirring frequently. Cook until mixture comes to a boil then add broth and tomatoes.

6. Cover skillet and cook for 90 minutes, take cover from pot and add bell pepper; cook for an additional 30 minutes or until thoroughly cooked.
7. Serve.

Nutritional Info

Calories 376

Carbs 37g

Fat 11g

Protein 25g

Beef Stroganoff

Serves: 1

Preparation Time: 45minutes

Ingredients

Olive oil (1 teaspoon)

Green beans (1 cup)

Garlic (1 clove, diced)

Cornstarch (1 teaspoon)

Worcestershire sauce (1 teaspoon)

Bell pepper (1 tablespoon, diced)

Black pepper

Mushrooms (1 ½ cups, sliced)

Onion (3/4 cup, diced)

Beef (2 oz., eye of round, sliced)

Beef broth (1/4 cup, no salt)

Tomato paste (1 teaspoon)

Yogurt (1/2 cup, low fat)

Directions

1. Heat ½ teaspoon oil in a skillet and sauté mushrooms, onions, garlic and green beans for 5 minutes until tender; take from pot and put aside.
2. Heat leftover oil in skillet and cook beef for 5 minutes then return vegetable mix to pot.
3. Combine broth, tomato paste, Worcestershire sauce and cornstarch until mixture is smooth.
4. Add mixture to beef along with bell peppers; cook for 10 minutes until sauce starts to bubble; add yogurt.
5. Top with parsley and serve.

Nutritional Info

Calories 340 Carbs 37g Fat 10g

Protein 30g

Chorizo and Black Bean Chili

Serves: 6

Preparation Time: 45minutes

Ingredients

Onions (2, diced)

Bell peppers (1 cup, red)

Butternut squash (1 cup, cubed)

Canned tomatoes (15 oz., diced)

Chili powder (2 tablespoons)

Smoked paprika (2 teaspoons)

Vegetable broth (4 cups, no salt)

Vegan Cheddar cheese (1 cup, shredded)

Bell peppers (2 cup, green, chopped)

Garlic (2 cloves, diced)

Canned black beans (15 oz., drained)

Jalapeno (1, diced)

Cumin (2 teaspoons)

Chipotle chorizo sausage (6 links)

Black pepper

Directions

1. Heat skillet and use cooking spray to coat then add garlic, bell peppers, onions and squash; cook for 5 minutes then add broth and cook for an additional 5 minutes.
2. Add all remaining ingredients and mix together to combine.
3. Cook for 10 minutes until chili comes to a boil and cook for an additional 15 minutes.
4. Serve.

Nutritional Info

Calories 372 Carbs 40g Fat 13g Protein 27g

Pork and Black Beans with Cauliflower and Broccoli

Serves: 4

Preparation Time: 45minutes

Ingredients

Onions (1 cup, diced)

Bell pepper (1, yellow, seeds remove and chopped)

Boneless pork (12 oz., fat removed and cubed)

Ground chipotle (1/2 teaspoon)

Liquid smoke (2 teaspoons)

Soy sauce (1 tablespoon, low salt)

Cauliflower (4 cups, florets)

Olive oil (1 tablespoon, extra- virgin)

Olives (24, pimento-stuffed, sliced)

Carrots (1/2 lb., cut in halves)

Canned tomatoes (14 oz., diced, no salt)

Cumin (1/2 teaspoon)

Garlic (2 cloves, diced)

Canned black beans (1 cup, drained)

Water (1 cup)

Broccoli (4 cups, florets)

Balsamic vinegar (2 ½ tablespoons)

Parsley (1/2 cup, chopped)

Directions

1.   Add all ingredients to slow cooker except soy sauce; stir to combine and cover.

2. Set on low and cook for 6-8 hours or on high for 3-4 hours.
3. Steam broccoli and cauliflower until crisp and tender.
4. Add soy sauce to stew, stir and serve with vegetables.

Nutritional Info

Calories 372

Carbs 40g

Fat 13g

Protein 27g

Braised Apple and Celery with Scallops

Serves: 1

Preparation Time: 15 minutes

Ingredients

Celery (3/4 cup, diced)

Vegetable broth (1/2 cup, no salt)

Ginger (1/2 teaspoon, grated)

Cardamom (1 teaspoon)

Olive oil (1 teaspoon)

Carrot (1/3 cup, shredded)

Green beans (1 cup)

Green apple (3/4, without core and chopped)

Scallops (4 oz.)

Walnuts (1 tablespoon, crushed)

Directions

1. Add carrots and celery to pot along with 3 tablespoon broth and cook for 5 minutes.
2. Put in leftover broth along with ginger, cardamom, green beans and apple; mix together to combine and cook until thoroughly heated.
3. Heat skillet and coat with cooking spray and cook scallops on all sides until golden.
4. Serve with vegetables and top with walnuts and olive oil.

Nutritional Info

Calories 324

Carbs 36g

Fat 11g

Protein 23g

Broccoli Casserole

Serves: 1

Preparation Time: 60 minutes

Ingredients

Broccoli (1 ½ cups, chopped)

Onions (1/2 cup, chopped)

Canned garbanzo beans (1/4 cup, drained)

Vegan mozzarella cheese (1/4 cup, shredded)

Olive oil (1/2 teaspoon)

Mushrooms (1 cup, chopped)

Bell pepper (1/2 cup, chopped)

Egg whites (1/2 cup)

Mayonnaise (1 teaspoon, light)

Almonds (2 teaspoons, silvered)

Directions

1. Set oven to 350°F.
2. Use cooking spray to coat a baking dish.
3. Add vegetables to dish and combine cheese, oil, egg whites and mayo in a bowl and pour over vegetables.
4. Top with almonds and bake for 35 minutes.
5. Serve.

Nutritional Info

Calories 350

Carbs 38g

Fat 11g

Protein 30g

Broccoli Orzo

Serves: 1

Preparation Time: 15 minutes

Ingredients

Orzo (1/3 cup)

Tomatoes (2 tablespoons, sun-dried, chopped)

Turmeric (1/4 teaspoon)

Lemon juice (1 tablespoon, freshly squeezed)

Broccoli (1 ½ cups)

Garlic powder (1/4 teaspoon)

Black pepper

Olive oil (1 ½ teaspoons, extra-virgin)

Directions

1. Prepare orzo as directed on package adding broccoli in final 3 minutes of cooking; remove from heat, drain and put aside. Reserve a ½ cup of cooking liquid.
2. Heat skillet and coat with cooking spray. Add orzo and leftover ingredients, stir and cook until thoroughly heated; add cooking liquid to avoid sticking.
3. Serve.

Nutritional Info

Calories 303

Carbs 34g

Fat 10g

Protein 20g

Broccoli and Ginger Chicken

Serves: 1

Preparation Time: 15 minutes

Ingredients

Chicken breast (3 oz., boneless and cut into strips)

Stir fry mix (1 ½ cups, snap peas and broccoli)

Onion (3/4 cup, chopped)

Water (1/4 cup)

Sesame oil (2 teaspoons)

Broccoli (1 ½ cups)

Water chestnuts (3 tablespoons, sliced)

Ginger (1 tablespoon, grated)

Soy sauce (1 tablespoon, low salt)

Directions

1. Heat oil in a wok or skillet and add chicken; cook for 5 minutes until meat is browned.
2. Add stir fry mix, onion, water, broccoli, chestnuts, soy sauce and ginger.
3. Stir mixture together and cook for 10 minutes or liquid has reduced. Do not allow all of liquid to evaporate, add more if necessary.
4. Serve.

Nutritional Info

Calories 344

Carbs 34g

Fat 10g

Protein 29g

Cajun Salmon

Serves: 1

Preparation Time: 30 minutes

Ingredients

Bell pepper (1/2 cup, sliced)

Salmon (3.5 oz.)

Broccoli (2 cups, chopped)

Onion (1/4 cup, sliced)

Cajun seasoning (1 teaspoon)

Olive oil (1 teaspoon, extra-virgin)

Directions

1. Set oven to 350F. Use foil to line a baking sheet and coat with cooking spray.
2. Coat onions and pepper with cooking spray and put onto prepare baking sheet. Coat salmon with Cajun seasoning and put onto sheet long with broccoli.
3. Bake for 25 minutes until fish is flaky.
4. Serve fish accompanied by vegetables; drizzle oil over vegetables if so desired.

Nutritional Info

Calories 353

Carbs 40g

Fat 12g

Protein 26g

Chicken Cordon Bleu

Serves: 2

Preparation Time: 35 minutes

Ingredients

Oat bran (6 teaspoons)

Agave nectar (1/2 teaspoon)

Ham slice (1 oz., halved)

Chicken broth (1/2 cup, no salt)

Greek yogurt (3 tablespoons, no fat)

Olive oil (1 tablespoon, extra-virgin)

Tomato (1, sliced)

Orange (1)

Dijon mustard (3 tablespoons)

Chicken breast (5 oz., boneless and skin removed)

Vegan Swiss cheese (1 oz., halved)

Broccoli (4 cups)

Apple (1)

Directions

1. Set oven to 375F.
2. Put 4 teaspoons of bran on a plate and put aside till needed. Combine agave and half of mustard in a small bowl.
3. Use mallet to pound meat until about ¼ inch thick. Top chicken breast with ham and cheese; roll and use a toothpick to hold in place.
4. Coat with agave mixture and then in bran. Use foil to line a baking sheet and coat with cooking spray.
5. Bake for 20 minutes. Place broccoli in a steamer and prepare sauce.
6. Combine 1 teaspoon of bran and stock in a saucepan, whisk until mixture is combined thoroughly; cook mixture until it gets thick then lower heat.

7. Add yogurt and leftover mustard, stir to combine and remove from heat.
8. Serve steamed broccoli with chicken and tomato. Top with sauce and garnish with apple and orange.

Nutritional Info

Calories 380

Carbs 39g

Fat 11g

Protein 32g

Chicken Kali

Serves: 1

Preparation Time: 30 minutes

Ingredients

Green beans (1 cup)

Chicken breast (3 oz., skinless and boneless)

Garlic (1 clove)

Curry powder (1 teaspoon)

Bell pepper (1, red)

Soy sauce (1 teaspoon, low salt)

Almonds (1 teaspoon, silvered)

Olive oil (1 ½ teaspoons)

Vidalia onion (1 cup, chopped)

Ginger (1 tablespoon, diced)

Mint (1 teaspoon, dried)

Chicken broth (2 tablespoons, no salt)

Mandarin (1/4 cup)

Directions

1. Steam green beans in a steamer or by preferred method.
2. Heat oil in a skillet and cook onion with chicken; add spices and stir to combine then add soy sauce and broth.
3. Cook for 15 minutes until thoroughly cooked then add mandarin and bell pepper; stir fry for 2 minutes.
4. Top with almond and serve with green beans.

Nutritional Info

Calories 345 Carbs 39g Fat 11g

Protein 25g

Chicken Apple Pie

Serves: 2

Preparation Time: 30 minutes

Ingredients

Broccoli (2 cups)

Cider vinegar (6 tablespoons)

Applesauce (3/4 cup, unsweetened)

Cinnamon (1/2 teaspoon)

Parsley (1/2 teaspoon)

Black pepper

Olive oil (3 teaspoons)

Chicken breast (6 oz., skinless and boneless)

Fruit cocktail (1 ½ cups, in water)

Mushrooms (5 cups, sliced)

Paprika (1/4 teaspoon)

Directions

1. Steam broccoli as preferred and put aside until needed.
2. Heat 1 teaspoon oil in a skillet and pound chicken until flattened then add to pot with 4 teaspoons of vinegar. Cook for 5 minutes until browned.
3. Add fruit cocktail, cinnamon and applesauce, stir to coat chicken and cook for 10 minutes.
4. Using another skillet heat leftover oil and sauté steamed broccoli and mushrooms with leftover vinegar; cook mushrooms until they are tender.
5. Serve chicken with sautéed vegetables. Top with paprika, black pepper and parsley.

Nutritional Info

Calories 319 Carbs 36g Fat 10g

Protein 27g

Chicken and Avocado Dip

Serves: 1

Preparation Time: 25 minutes

Ingredients

Avocado (1/2)

Lime juice (1 tablespoon, freshly squeezed)

Baby spinach (3 cups)

Red onion (2 slices)

Brussels sprouts (1 cup, cooked)

Mango (1/3 cup, ripe)

Chicken breast (3 oz.)

Mrs. Dash seasoning

Mushrooms (1 cup)

Herb dressing (2 tablespoons)

Olive oil (1/2 teaspoon)

Directions

1. Put lime juice, mango and avocado into a blender or processor and blend together.
2. Use Mrs. Dash seasoning to season chicken breast and place on a grill for 15 minutes until thoroughly cooked.
3. Place chicken onto a plate and top with avocado dip.
4. Heat skillet and coat with cooking spray then add mushrooms and sauté for 5 minutes then add spinach and cook for 3 minutes or until wilted.
5. Add spinach and mushroom to plate and top with dressing; add sprouts and drizzle with oil.
6. Serve.

Nutritional Info

Calories 358 Carbs 39g Fat 10g

Protein 36g

Chicken Radicchio Salad

Serves: 2

Preparation Time: 25 minutes

Ingredients

Chicken breast (5 oz., sliced)

Prosciutto (2 oz.)

Balsamic vinegar (2 tablespoons)

Blueberries (1/2 cup)

Peaches (2, pits removed and sliced)

Radicchio (2 cups)

Almonds (2 tablespoon, toasted)

Strawberries (1 cup)

Directions

1. Set oven to 350℉.
2. Place chicken breast in a baking dish and top with prosciutto and radicchio; bake for 15 minutes.
3. Drizzle vinegar on top of baked chicken.
4. Top with almonds, peach and berries.
5. Serve.

Nutritional Info

Calories 336

Carbs 32g

Fat 11g

Protein 27g

Shrimp and Chickpeas Mexicali

Serves: 2

Preparation Time: 20 minutes plus chilling time

Ingredients

Olive oil (1 tablespoon)

Jalapeno (1, diced without seeds)

Garlic (1 clove, diced)

Lime juice (3 tablespoons, freshly squeezed)

Canned garbanzo beans (1/2 cup, drained)

Shrimp (7 oz., cooked)

Chipotle (2 tablespoons, in adobo sauce, chopped)

Red onion (1 cup, chopped)

Tomato (3 cups, chopped)

Cilantro (1/4 cup, chopped)

Directions

1. Put chipotle, red onion, garlic, olive oil and jalapeno in a bowl; whisk together until thoroughly combined.
2. Add lime juice, beans, tomato and cilantro to mixture and toss to combine.
3. Adjust seasonings to desired taste and chill for at least 2 hours.
4. Serve topped with shrimp.

Nutritional Info

Calories 357

Carbs 38g

Fat 11g

Protein 28g

Chinese Orzo

Serves: 1

Preparation Time: 20 minutes

Ingredients

Orzo pasta (1/3 cup)

Egg whites (2)

Garlic (1 clove)

Olive oil (1/2 teaspoon)

Frozen vegetable mix (1 ½ cups, broccoli, sugar snap peas, chestnuts and carrots)

Scallion (2 tablespoons, chopped)

Soy sauce (1 teaspoon, low salt)

Sesame oil (1 teaspoon, toasted)

Directions

1. Prepare orzo as directed on package, drain and run under cold water, drain again and put aside.
2. Prepare frozen vegetable mix as directed on package and put with orzo.
3. Heat oil olive and sesame oil in a skillet and sauté garlic and scallion. Add egg whites to pot and scramble.
4. Add cooked vegetables and orzo and toss to combine; heat mixture thoroughly.
5. Serve.

Nutritional Info

Calories 337

Carbs 32g

Fat 10g

Protein 25g

Green Beans and Chorizo

Serves: 2

Preparation Time: 45 minutes

Ingredients

Vegetable broth (2 tablespoons, unsalted)

Canned tomatoes (14.5 oz., stewed)

Garlic (1 clove)

Cumin (1/4 teaspoon)

Chorizo chicken sausage (3 links, chipotle flavor)

Mushrooms (2 cups, sliced)

Green beans (2 cups)

Chili powder (1/2 teaspoon)

Cayenne pepper (1/4 teaspoon)

Peaches (2)

Directions

1. Prepare orzo as directed on package, drain and run under cold water, drain again and put aside.
2. Prepare frozen vegetable mix as directed on package and put with orzo.
3. Heat oil olive and sesame oil in a skillet and sauté garlic and scallion. Add egg whites to pot and scramble.
4. Add cooked vegetables and orzo and toss to combine; heat mixture thoroughly.
5. Serve.

Nutritional Info

Calories 358

Carbs 41g

Fat 12g

Protein 30g

Three Bean Salad and Chicken Marinara

Serves: 1

Preparation Time: 40 minutes

Ingredients

Green beans (1 ½ cups, cut in halves)

Canned kidney beans (1/4 cup, drained)

Cider vinegar (2 tablespoons)

Parsley (1 teaspoon, dried)

Basil (1 ½ teaspoons, dried)

Tomato and basil sauce (1/4 cup)

Vegan mozzarella cheese (3 tablespoons, shredded)

Canned garbanzo beans (1/4 cup, drained)

Olive oil (1 teaspoon)

Chives (1 teaspoon, dried)

Black pepper (1/2 teaspoon)

Chicken breast (3 oz.)

Garlic powder (1/2 teaspoon)

Directions

1. Set oven to 450°F.
2. Steam green beans until crisp preferably in a steamer. Combine green beans with kidney and chickpeas in a bowl.
3. In a small bowl add oil, chives, black pepper, vinegar, 1 teaspoon basil and parsley; whisk together and add to beans mixture. Toss to combine and chill for 30 minutes or until ready to serve.
4. Put chicken onto a piece of foil (large enough to wrap chicken). Add tomato sauce to chicken along with garlic powder, cheese and leftover basil.
5. Wrap chicken leaving a small opening. Place foil on a baking tray and bake for 20 minutes.
6. Serve chicken with bean salad.

Nutritional Info

Calories 368 Carbs 40g Fat 12g

Protein 29g

Crab Bisque

Serves: 1

Preparation Time: 60 minutes

Ingredients

Onion (1/4 cup, chopped)

Cornstarch (1 teaspoon)

Crab (4 oz.)

Cauli-mash (1 cup) - recipe above

Olive oil (1 teaspoon)

Coconut milk (3/4 cup)

Black pepper

Fish seasoning (1 teaspoon)

Directions

1. Heat oil in a soup pot and cook onion for 3 minutes until soft and clear.
2. Combine milk with cornstarch and add to pot. Heat mixture until it gets thick; add fish seasoning and stir to combine.
3. Add crab and cook until thoroughly heated.
4. Serve with cauli-mash.

Nutritional Info

Calories 339

Carbs 35g

Fat 9g

Protein 32g

Curried Eggplant

Serves: 1

Preparation Time: 60 minutes

Ingredients

Turkey breast (3 oz., ground)

Eggplant (1 cup, peel removed and diced)

Mushrooms (1 cup, sliced)

Red curry paste (1 tablespoon)

Olive oil (2 teaspoons)

Onion (1/2 cup, chopped)

Canned tomatoes (1 ½ cups, diced with liquid)

Directions

1. Heat oil in a deep skillet and cook turkey for 10 minutes until browned all over.
2. Add vegetables and curry paste to pot, stir to combine and cover pot.
3. Cook over a low flame for 45 minutes, stir occasionally to avoid sticking.
4. Serve.

Nutritional Info

Calories 339

Carbs 35g

Fat 9g

Protein 32g

Lime and Dill Salmon

Serves: 1

Preparation Time: 30 minutes

Ingredients

Zucchini (1/4 lb., sliced)

Onion (1/2, sliced into rings)

Olive oil (1/2 teaspoon)

Italian seasoning (1 teaspoon)

Sparkling water (1 ½ cups, lime flavor, no sugar added)

Onion powder (1 teaspoon)

Salmon (4 oz.)

Summer squash (1/4 lb., sliced)

Tomatoes (2, sliced)

Black pepper

Dill weed (1 tablespoon)

Brussels sprouts (1 cup, frozen)

Directions

1. Slice vegetables and place onto a large piece of foil. Use oil to coat vegetables, top with spices and wrap foil around vegetables.
2. Place foil on a grill and cook vegetables or bake in an oven at 350F for 25 minutes.
3. Heat seasoning and water in a skillet, put in salmon and poach for 3 minutes. Use liquid to coat fish and flip fish, cook for 4 minutes on the other side.
4. Prepare sprouts as directed on package.
5. Serve salmon with sprouts and vegetables.

Nutritional Info

Calories 369 Carbs 43g Fat 10g

Protein 34g

Cabbage Soup

Serves: 2

Preparation Time: 45 minutes

Ingredients

Olive oil (2 teaspoons)

Onions (3/4 cup, chopped)

Cabbage (4 cups, shredded)

Bell peppers (1 ½ cups, diced)

Garlic (2 cloves, diced)

Tabasco sauce (1/8 teaspoon)

Ground turkey (6 oz.)

Canned garbanzo beans (1/3 cup, drained)

Mushrooms (1 ½ cups, sliced)

Tomatoes (1 ¼ cups, chopped)

Caraway seeds (1/8 teaspoon)

Black pepper

Vegetable broth (4 cups, unsalted)

Extra olive oil (for drizzle)

Directions

1. Heat oil in a skillet and sauté onions then add turkey and cook for 10 minutes until browned.
2. Add remaining ingredients, stir to combine and cover pot; cook for 30 minutes.
3. Serve topped with olive oil.

Nutritional Info

Calories 366 Carbs 40g

Fat 11g

Protein 29g

Chicken Eggplant Parmigiana

Serves: 2

Preparation Time: 50 minutes

Ingredients

Olive oil (3 teaspoons)

Eggplant (3 cups, diced)

Chicken breast (5 oz., sliced in half)

Vegan mozzarella cheese (1/3 cups, shredded)

Cornmeal (1 tablespoon)

Onion (2 cups, chopped)

Tomato (1, chopped)

Tomato sauce (3/4cup, no sugar or salt)

Breadcrumbs (1 tablespoon)

Grapes (1/3 cup)

Directions

1. Set oven to 350F.
2. Heat 2 teaspoons oil in a skillet and cook onions for 3 minutes until clear; put in eggplant and cook for 10 minutes until soft.
3. Add chicken, tomato and cook for an additional 10 minutes.
4. Use tomato sauce to cover bottom of casserole dish and then add cooked eggplant and chicken. Top with cornmeal and breadcrumbs then with the cheese and leftover oil.
5. Bake for 15 minutes then broil for an additional 5 minutes.
6. Serve warm.

Nutritional Info

Calories 360

Carbs 40g

Fat 13g

Protein 25g

Grill Bluefish

Serves: 3

Preparation Time: 2 hours

Ingredients

Red onion (2 tablespoons)

Lemon juice (2 tablespoon, freshly squeezed)

Jalapeno pepper (1/2, seeds removed and diced)

Bluefish fillets (4 oz.)

Lemon (2 tablespoons, with seeds or membrane, chopped)

Olive oil (1 teaspoon)

Asparagus (2 cups)

All-purpose seasoning (1/4 teaspoon)

Directions

1. Combine red onion, lemon juice, jalapeno, lemon and olive oil in a small bowl; steam asparagus.
2. Use seasoning to season fish and heat skillet. Coat with cooking spray and cook for 4 minutes on each side.
3. Serve fish with steamed asparagus and lemon salsa.

Nutritional Info

Calories 334

Carbs 38g

Fat 10g

Protein 30g

Eggplant Parmesan

Serves: 1

Preparation Time: 20 minutes

Ingredients

Olive oil (1 teaspoon)

Garlic (1 clove, diced)

Breadcrumbs (2 teaspoons)

Oregano (1/2 teaspoon)

Tomato sauce (1 cup)

Vegan mozzarella (1/4 cup, shredded)

Egg whites (3)

Vegan Parmesan (2 teaspoons)

Basil (1 teaspoon)

Black pepper (1/2 teaspoon)

Eggplant (1 ½ cups, cubed)

Directions

1. Set oven to 350°F.
2. Heat oil in a deep skillet.
3. Add garlic, crumbs, oregano, tomato sauce, egg whites, parmesan, basil, black pepper and eggplant to a bowl. Mix together and add to skillet; cook for 5 minutes.
4. Coat a baking dish with cooking spray and transfer eggplant mixture to dish.
5. Top with mozzarella and bake for 10 minutes.
6. Serve warm.

Nutritional Info

Calories 341 Carbs 37g

Fat 12g

Protein 27g

Creamy Spicy Chicken Stew

Serves: 6

Preparation Time: 10 hours

Ingredients

Chicken breasts (20 oz., without skin and bones)

Canned tomatoes (40 oz., diced with juices)

Canned black beans (3/4 cup, drained)

Green beans (10 oz.)

Cilantro (1 tablespoon, chopped)

Cumin (1 teaspoon)

Olive oil (2 tablespoons, extra-virgin)

Onion (1 ½ cups, chopped)

Green salsa (16 oz.)

Canned pinto beans (15 oz., drained)

Taco seasoning (1.25 oz.)

Chili pepper (2 teaspoons)

Cream cheese (4 oz., low fat, soft)

Directions

1. Add onions and chicken to a slow cooker and top with tomatoes, black beans, green beans, salsa and pinto.
2. Stir to combine and add taco seasoning, chili, cumin and cilantro.
3. Set cooker on low and cook for 8-10 hours until mixture is slightly thickened but not too thick.
4. Take 2 tablespoons of stew from pot and combine with cream cheese until smooth then add to stew and mix together; cook for 15 minutes more.
5. Serve topped with olive oil.

Nutritional Info

Calories 341 Carbs 37g Fat 12g Protein 27g

Roasted Vegetables and Fusilli

Serves: 1

Preparation Time: 25 minutes

Ingredients

Fusilli (3/4 cup)

Roma tomatoes (3, cut in halves)

Garlic (2 cloves with peel)

Curry

Olive oil (1 teaspoon)

Eggplant (1 cup, cubed)

Feta cheese (2 tablespoons)

Herb seasoning

Basil (1 tablespoon, chopped)

Directions

1. Set oven to 425°F.
2. Put garlic, eggplant and tomatoes onto a baking sheet and coat with cooking spray, black pepper and herb seasoning; bake for 20 minutes.
3. While vegetables are roasting, prepare fusilli as directed on package and drain; aside till needed.
4. Take roasted vegetables from oven and squeeze garlic out of peel into a bowl. Add pasta, roasted vegetables, basil, cheese and oil.
5. Toss and serve. May be chilled.

Nutritional Info

Calories 318

Carbs 35g

Fat 10g

Protein 21g

Shrimp Fusilli with Asparagus and Roasted Tomatoes

Serves: 1

Preparation Time: 40 minutes

Ingredients

Fusilli (3/4 cup)

Roma tomatoes (3, cut in halves)

Asparagus (1 ½ cups, trimmed and cut in halves)

Garlic (3 cloves with peel)

Shrimp (4, deveined and peeled)

Lemon juice (1/2 teaspoon, freshly squeezed)

Thyme (1/8 teaspoon)

Olive oil (1 ½ teaspoons)

Oregano (1/4 teaspoon)

Directions

1. Set oven to 375°F.
2. Put garlic and tomatoes in a roasting pan and coat with cooking spray and black pepper. Roast for 15 minutes until tomatoes wrinkle.
3. Add shrimp and asparagus on top of roasted tomatoes and bake for 10 minutes. Take garlic from pan and remove peel; put aside to cool for 5 minutes and cover pan to keep warm.
4. Prepare fusilli as directed on package. While pasta cooks, mash garlic in a bowl.
5. Drain pasta, saving ½ cup of cooking liquid and put aside till needed.
6. Heat oil in a pan then add mashed garlic, oregano, lemon juice and thyme. Toss to combine, adding reserved liquid to avoid sticking.
7. Serve topped with tomatoes, shrimp and asparagus.

Nutritional Info

Calories 347

Carbs 37g

Fat 11g

Protein 27g

Grilled Sole Filet and Leeks

Serves: 1

Preparation Time: 40 minutes

Ingredients

Olive oil (2 teaspoons)

Sole filet (4.5 oz.)

Garlic (1 teaspoon, diced)

Dill (1 teaspoon, fresh)

Lemon-herb seasoning (1/2 teaspoon)

Leeks (1 cup, sliced)

White wine (4 oz.)

Shallot (1 tablespoon, diced)

Black pepper

Directions

1. Set oven to 375F.
2. Coat a baking dish with cooking spray and place leeks into dish and top with filet.
3. Put wine, shallots, black pepper, garlic and dill in a bowl; whisk together and pour on top of sole.
4. Add herb seasoning, cover dish and bake for 30 minutes.
5. Serve.

Nutritional Info

Calories 394

Carbs 29g

Fat 11g

Protein 26g

Turkey and Mandarin Salad

Serves: 1

Preparation Time: 15 minutes

Ingredients

Turkey breast (3 oz., cooked, cut into cubes)

Red onion (3/4 cup, diced)

French dressing (3 tablespoons)

Mandarin orange (1/3 cup)

Mint (1 tablespoon, fresh, chopped)

Baby spinach (1 cup)

Celery (1 cup, diced)

Olive oil (2 teaspoons)

Peach (1, pit removed and sliced)

Turmeric (1/8 teaspoon)

Romaine lettuce (1 cup, chopped)

Directions

1. Add celery, oil, peach, turmeric, mint, turkey, onion, dressing and oranges to a bowl; toss to combine.
2. Arrange spinach and lettuce on a dish and top with turkey mixture.
3. Serve. May be chilled.

Nutritional Info

Calories 378

Carbs 42g

Fat 11g

Protein 31g

Vegetable Beef Soup

Serves: 4

Preparation Time: 60 minutes

Ingredients

Ground beef (12 oz., lean)

Carrots (1 cup, sliced)

Canned garbanzo beans (1 cup)

Tomato puree (1/2 cup)

Beef broth (4 cups, no salt)

Peppercorns (4)

Marjoram (1/2 teaspoon)

Chives (1/4 teaspoon)

Oregano (1/2 teaspoon)

Celery (2 ½ cups, diced)

Onion (1 cup, chopped)

Tomatoes (2 cups, chopped)

Olive oil (1 ½ tablespoons)

Garlic (4 cloves, crushed)

Worcestershire sauce (1/2 teaspoon)

Parsley (1 teaspoon)

Directions

1. Heat oil in a large and add garlic, onion and tomatoes; cook for 5 minutes then add beef and cook for 5 minutes until slightly golden. Add all remaining ingredients and stir.
2. Bring mixture to a boil, cover pot and cook for 40 minutes till vegetables are cooked.

Nutritional Info

Calories 357 Carbs 39g

Fat 11g

Protein 29g

Asian Style Halibut

Serves: 4

Preparation Time: 30 minutes

Ingredients

Bok Choy (8 cups, chopped)

Halibut filets (4)

Scallions (3, chopped)

Soy sauce (3 tablespoons, low salt)

Sesame oil (1 ½ teaspoons)

Cauliflower (6 cups)

Sweet potatoes (2, washed with peel)

Red bell pepper (1, sliced thin)

Black pepper (1/2 teaspoon)

Orange zest (1 tablespoon)

Rice vinegar (1 ½ teaspoons)

Ginger (1 tablespoon, grated)

Olive oil (4 teaspoons)

Directions

1. Set oven to 400F.
2. Lay a piece foil that can wrap a filet. Put bell pepper and bok choy onto foil, add filet and top with scallion, zest and black pepper. Repeat with remaining filets.
3. Add vinegar, ginger, soy sauce and sesame oil to a bowl, whisk together and add to filets in foil. Wrap foil and fish and bake for 15 minutes.
4. Steam cauliflower while fish cooks. Use a fork to pierce potatoes all over and microwave for 4 minutes, turn over and cook for an additional 4 minutes.
5. Serve fish with potato and cauliflower. Drizzle with olive oil.

Nutritional Info

Calories 364 Carbs 39g Fat 10g Protein 32g

Stir Fry Hot & Sour Pork with Cabbage

Serves: 1

Preparation Time: 60 minutes

Ingredients

Olive oil (1 ½ teaspoons)

Cornstarch (1 teaspoon)

Cider vinegar (1 tablespoon)

Garlic (2 teaspoons, diced)

Pork loin (3 oz., cut up large)

Onion (1/2 cup, sliced)

Bell pepper (1, red, sliced thin)

Vegetable broth (1/2 cup)

Soy sauce (1 tablespoon, low salt)

Scallions (1/2 cup, chopped)

Ginger (2 teaspoons, diced)

Cauliflower (1 cup, florets)

Cabbage (2 cups, shredded)

Jalapeno (2 tablespoons, chopped)

Directions

1. Add ginger, garlic, scallions, vinegar, soy sauce, cornstarch, broth and oil to a bowl. Whisk together and add pork to mixture. Cover bowl and place in fridge for 30 minutes.
2. Heat a skillet and coat with cooking spray. Add pork to pot and cook for 20 minutes until meat is browned.
3. Add vegetables, stir to combine and cook for 5-10 minutes until vegetables are cooked.
4. Serve.

Nutritional Info

Calories 357 Carbs 38g

Fat 11g

Protein 27

Shrimp, Yogurt and Apples Salad

Serves: 1

Preparation Time: 20 minutes

Ingredients

Ginger (1/8 teaspoon, diced)

Cilantro (1 tablespoon)

Turmeric (1/4 teaspoon)

Cumin (1/8 teaspoon)

Soy yogurt (1/2 cup, low fat)

Onion (1/2 cup, diced)

Shrimp (4 oz., small, deveined and shell removed)

Garlic (1 clove, diced)

Tabasco sauce (1/4 teaspoon)

Coriander (1/8 teaspoon)

Cider vinegar (2 teaspoons)

Apple (1/2)

Romaine lettuce (3 cups, chopped)

Directions

1. Heat oil in a skillet and add garlic, onions, cilantro, coriander and cook for 3 minutes then add shrimp and remaining spices. Stir to combine and cook for 2minutes.
2. Heat yogurt, onion, vinegar and apple in a small saucepan and add to shrimp. Toss to combine.
3. Serve shrimp on top of lettuce.

Nutritional Info

Calories 325 Carbs 33g

Fat 11g

Protein 26g

Lentils and Italian Beef

Serves: 2

Preparation Time: 30 minutes

Ingredients

Onion (1/2 cup, chopped)

Bay leaves (2)

Ground beef (7 oz., lean)

Lentils (1 cup, cooked)

Italian seasoning

Olive oil (1 ½ teaspoons, extra virgin)

Celery (1/2 cup, chopped)

Garlic (2 cloves, crushed)

Canned tomatoes (14.5 oz., diced)

Black pepper

Directions

1. Heat oil in a skillet and add bay leaves, celery and onion for 3 minutes until soft and translucent.
2. Add garlic and beef and cook for 15 minutes until beef is golden all over. Put in tomatoes and lentils and cook for 5 minutes until thoroughly heated.
3. Add black pepper and Italian seasoning; stir to combine.
4. Serve.

Nutritional Info

Calories 325

Carbs 33g

Fat 11g

Protein 26g

Noodle-free Lasagna

Serves: 1

Preparation Time: 50 minutes

Ingredients

Oregano (1/2 teaspoon)

Olive oil (1 ½ teaspoons)

Tofu (1/4 cup, firm, cubed)

Asparagus (1 cup, chopped)

Mushrooms (1/2 cup, chopped)

Spinach (1 cup)

Canned tomatoes (14.5 oz., diced)

Basil (1/2 teaspoon)

Egg whites (2/3 cup)

Ricotta cheese (2 tablespoons, low fat)

Red pepper (1/3 cup, roasted, chopped)

Zucchini (1 cup, chopped)

Vegan mozzarella (2 teaspoons, shredded)

Directions

1. Set oven to 350F.
2. Combine Italian seasoning and tomatoes in a bowl; reserve 4 tablespoons aside.
3. Heat skillet and coat with cooking spray. Combine egg whites and 1 teaspoon oil and add to pot, swirl around pot until it spreads to form a thin layer. Cut the egg to fit your baking dish.
4. Add tofu, asparagus, mushrooms, ricotta, zucchini and peppers to seasoned tomatoes and combine.
5. Arrange 'lasagna' by adding a layer of egg whites to dish then add tomato mixture and spinach. Finish layering lasagna with leftover ingredients. Top with reserved tomatoes and cheese.

6. Bake for 40 minutes.
7. Cool and serve topped with leftover oil.

.Nutritional Info

Calories 371

Carbs 44g

Fat 11g

Protein 35g

Beef and Vegetable Stir Fry

Serves: 1

Preparation Time: 15 minutes (plus marinating time)

Ingredients

Red wine (2 tablespoons, dry)

Worcestershire sauce (2 teaspoons)

Basil (1 tablespoon, chopped)

Parsley (1 tablespoon, chopped)

Beef (3 oz., cubed)

Bell pepper (1/2, green)

Yellow squash (1/2 cup, cubed)

Tomato (3/4, chopped)

Olive oil (1/2 teaspoon)

Balsamic vinegar (1 ½ tablespoons)

Garlic (2 teaspoons, diced)

Mint (1 tablespoon, chopped)

Black pepper

Bell pepper (1/2, red)

Zucchini (2 cups, cubed)

Mushrooms (1 cup, sliced)

Directions

1. Add vinegar, garlic, mint, black pepper, 1 teaspoon oil, Worcestershire sauce, basil and parsley to a bowl and mix together.
2. Put meat into mixture and coat; cover and place in refrigerator for 4 hours or overnight if preferred.

3. Slice up zucchini, mushrooms, tomatoes, pepper and squash. Heat a skillet and coat with cooking spray; add beef to pot and cook beef for 10 minutes then add vegetables and cook for an additional 5 minutes or until veggies are tender.
4. Serve.

Nutritional Info

Calories 347

Carbs 36g

Fat 10g

Protein 27g

Seafood Chowder

Serves: 2

Preparation Time: 25 minutes

Ingredients

Olive oil (1 tablespoon)

Water chestnuts (1/3 cup, chopped)

Parsley (1 tablespoon, chopped)

Worcestershire sauce (1/2 teaspoon)

Shrimp (3 oz., jumbo, diced)

Garlic (1 clove, chopped)

Coconut milk (1 cup)

Cornstarch (2 teaspoons)

Onions (1 cup, diced)

Celery (1 cup, diced)

Cilantro (1 tablespoon)

Hot sauce (1/2 teaspoon)

Scallops (4 oz., chopped)

Tomatoes (2, chopped)

Chicken broth (1 cup)

Water (1 cup)

Directions

1. Heat oil in a skillet and add onion, celery, cilantro, hot sauce, chestnuts, parsley and Worcestershire sauce; cook for 5 minutes until celery and onion are tender.
2. Add garlic, scallops and shrimp and cook for 5 minutes more until shrimp is pink.
3. Add broth to a small pot along with tomatoes, pre-cooked seafood mix and water; cook for 7 minutes then add coconut milk and cook for an additional 3 minutes.

4. Combine starch and some liquid from pot and add to pot. Stir to combine and cook until chowder gets thick.
5. Serve.

Nutritional Info

Calories 328

Carbs 36g

Fat 10g

Protein 26g

Gumbo

Serves: 2

Preparation Time: 40 minutes

Ingredients

Olive oil (2 teaspoons)

Onions (1 cup, chopped)

Bell pepper (1, chopped)

Vegetable broth (2 cups)

Cumin (1 teaspoon)

Thyme (1 teaspoon)

Old Bay seasoning (2 teaspoons)

Canned black beans (1/2 cup, drained)

Chorizo chicken sausage (1 link, sliced)

Okra (2 cups)

Garlic (3 cloves, diced)

Celery (1 cup, chopped)

Plum tomatoes (1 ½ cups, chopped)

Chili powder (2 teaspoons)

Bay leaf (1/2 teaspoon)

Filé powder (1 tablespoon)

Scallions (3, chopped)

Shrimp (4 oz., jumbo, cooked)

Directions

1. Heat oil in a soup pot and sauté okra for 3 minutes or until slightly golden.

2. Add garlic, celery, onion and pepper to pot and cook for 3 minutes more. Put in broth, cumin, thyme, Old Bay seasoning, black beans, tomatoes, chili powder, bay leaf and filé powder; cook for 25 minutes.
3. Add shrimp, sausage and scallions and cook for an additional 5 minutes.
4. Serve.

Nutritional Info

Calories 320

Carbs 33g

Fat 8g

Protein 28g

Meatloaf and Cheesy Veggies

Serves: 4

Preparation Time: 60 minutes

Ingredients

Egg whites (2)

Italian seasoning (1 tablespoon)

Garlic powder (3/4 teaspoon)

Soy sauce (1 tablespoon)

Steel cut oats (3 tablespoons, raw)

Celery (1/2 cup, diced)

Broccoli (2 cups)

Cauliflower (2 cups)

Vegan cheddar (1/2cup, shredded)

Canned kidney beans (1/2 cup, drained)

Onion flakes (2 tablespoons)

Red pepper (1/2 teaspoon)

Ground turkey (10 oz.)

Bell pepper (3/4 cup, diced)

Tomato sauce (1 cup)

Chives (1 tablespoon, dried)

Olive oil (1 tablespoon)

Directions

1. Set oven to 350F. Use cooking spray to coat a loaf pan.
2. Mix together beans, soy sauce, eggs and spices in a blender then pour into a large bowl.

3. Add oats, bell pepper, half of tomato sauce, meat, onion flakes and celery. Use hands to combine mixture and put into loaf pan. Spread leftover tomato sauce on top.
4. Bake for 60 minutes until loaf is set. Steam broccoli and cauliflower and add cheese and chives; cover pan and bake for an additional 3 minutes.
5. Slice loaf evenly and serve with veggies. Drizzle veggies with oil.

Nutritional Info

Calories 320

Carbs 33g

Fat 8g

Protein 28g

Cashew Orange Chicken

Serves: 2

Preparation Time: 60 minutes

Ingredients

Orange juice (1/3 cup)

Olive oil (1 ½ teaspoons)

Chicken breast (6 oz., boneless, cubed)

Cornstarch (1 ½ teaspoons)

Cashew nuts (2 teaspoons)

Soy sauce (2 tablespoons)

Ginger (1/2 teaspoon)

Mandarin orange (1 cup)

Green beans (2 cups)

Directions

1. Combine soy sauce, ginger, orange juice and half of oil in a bowl; add chicken to mixture and coat. Marinate for 30 minutes at room temperature.
2. Heat leftover oil in a skillet and cook chicken for 15 minutes until thoroughly cooked.
3. Combine cornstarch and leftover marinade. Add to chicken, stir to combine and cook until thick then add cashews and mandarin and cook until thoroughly heated.
4. Serve with green beans.

Nutritional Info

Calories 326

Carbs 35g

Fat 11g

Protein 24g

Herbed Orange Chicken

Serves: 1

Preparation Time: 20 minutes

Ingredients

Olive oil (1 teaspoon)

Cider vinegar (1 tablespoon)

Garlic (1 clove, chopped)

Onion (1/2 cup, chopped)

Orange juice (1/4 cup, freshly squeezed)

Mandarin (1/2 cup)

Brussels sprouts (1/2 cup)

Chicken breast (3 oz., diced)

Parsley (1 tablespoon, chopped)

Mushrooms (3 cups, sliced)

Water (2 tablespoons)

Orange extract (1/2 teaspoon)

Olive oil (1 teaspoon)

Directions

1. Heat half of oil in skillet and add garlic, parsley, chicken and vinegar; cook for 10 minutes.
2. While chicken cooks, heat leftover oil in another skillet and sauté mushrooms and onion for 5 minutes.
3. Add mandarin, orange juice and water to chicken and cook for 3 minutes; prepare sprouts.
4. Serve chicken with sprouts and mushrooms mixture.

Nutritional Info

Calories 361 Carbs 39g Fat 13g Protein 29g

Snow Peas and Oriental Turkey

Serves: 2

Preparation Time: 20 minutes

Ingredients

Olive oil (3 teaspoons)

Bean sprouts (2 cups)

Snow peas (3/4 cup)

Broccoli (3 cups, florets)

Worcestershire sauce (1 teaspoon)

Espagnol sauce (3/4 cup)

Ground turkey (6 oz.)

Bell pepper (2 cups, cut into strips)

Pearl onions (3/4 cup)

Soy sauce (1 teaspoon)

Balsamic vinegar (1 tablespoon)

Directions

1. Heat a teaspoon of oil in a skillet and cook bean sprouts and turkey for 10 minutes using spoon to break up meat as it cooks.
2. Heat leftover oil in another skillet and cook snow peas, broccoli, peppers, onions, vinegar, soy sauce and Worcestershire sauce for 5 minutes.
3. Add espagnol sauce to vegetables and mix together. Combine turkey and vegetable mixture.
4. Serve.

Nutritional Info

Calories 330 Carbs 36g

Fat 8g

Protein 32g

Baked Overstuffed Portobello Mushroom

Serves: 1

Preparation Time: 45 minutes

Ingredients

Portobello mushrooms (1, stem removed and diced)

Mushrooms (1 cup, chopped)

Celery (1/4 cup, chopped)

Bell peppers (1/4 cup, chopped)

Tomato (1, chopped)

Vegan mozzarella (1/4 cup, shredded)

Olive oil (1 teaspoon, extra-virgin)

Onion (1/2 cup, chopped)

Zucchini (1, chopped)

Garlic (1 clove, crushed)

Lentils (1/4 cup, cooked and crushed)

Egg whites (1/2 cup)

Directions

1. Set oven to 400F.
2. Heat a large skillet and coat with cooking spray. Add onion, zucchini, garlic, mushrooms, celery and peppers and cook for 8 minutes until tender; add tomatoes to mixture.
3. Place Portobello into a greased baking pan. Bake for 5 minutes until slightly tender.
4. Add lentils, 2 tablespoons of cheese and egg whites to vegetables; stir to combine.
5. Take Portobello from oven and fill with vegetable mixture, return stuffed Portobello to oven and bake for 15 minutes. Remove Portobello from oven, add cheese and bake for an additional 5 minutes.
6. Serve topped with a drizzle of oil.

Nutritional Info

Calories 356 Carbs 42g Fat 10g Protein 30g

Papered Fish

Serves: 1

Preparation Time: 30 minutes

Ingredients

White fish (4.5 oz.)

Onions (3/4 cup, chopped)

Olives (3, sliced)

Prickly pear (1/4 cup)

Black pepper

Bell pepper (1, red, sliced)

Mushrooms (5, sliced)

Olive oil (1 ½ teaspoons)

Mustard (1 tablespoon)

Green beans (1 cup)

Directions

1. Set oven to 425F.
2. Place half of olives and veggies on a piece of foil large enough to be wrapped. Coat fish with mustard and top with veggies and 1 teaspoon oil.
3. Wrap up foil and place on a baking sheet; bake for 15 minutes until fish is thoroughly cooked; boil green beans.
4. Serve beans with fish and veggies. Drizzle oil over beans.

Nutritional Info

Calories 366

Carbs 40g

Fat 11g

Protein 31g

Peking Shrimp

Serves: 2

Preparation Time: 15 minutes

Ingredients

Chicken broth (1/2 cup, no salt)

Cornstarch (4 teaspoons)

Garlic (1 tablespoon, diced)

Canned chestnuts (1/2 cup, drained and chopped)

Roasted peanuts (12, crushed)

Soy sauce (4 tablespoons, low salt)

Olive oil (1 tablespoon)

Stir fry vegetables (16 oz., snap peas mix)

Shrimp (8 oz., peel removed and deveined)

Apples (1, sliced)

Directions

1. Combine cornstarch, soy sauce and broth in a bowl; put aside until needed.
2. Heat half of oil in a skillet and add chestnuts, vegetables and garlic to the pot; cook for 3 minutes and put aside in a bowl.
3. Heat leftover oil and stir fry shrimp for 4 minutes then add cooked veggies to the pot. Add cornstarch mixture to shrimp and cook until it is bubbly.
4. Serve shrimp mix topped with apple and peanuts.

Nutritional Info

Calories 380

Carbs 31g

Fat 12g

Protein 32g

Poached Flounder

Serves: 2

Preparation Time: 30 minutes

Ingredients

Olive oil (1 teaspoon)

Flounder (8 oz.)

Old Bay seasoning (1/4 teaspoon)

Oregano (1 teaspoon)

Spinach (3 cups, cooked)

Olive oil (2 teaspoons)

Garlic (2 cloves, chopped)

Parsley (1 tablespoon)

White wine vinegar (1 tablespoon)

Directions

1. Heat oil in a skillet.
2. Coat flounder with Old Bay seasoning and add to pot. Top with parsley and add water and half of vinegar; cook for 10 minutes.
3. Drizzle spinach with leftover vinegar.
4. Serve. May be paired with Cauli-mash.

Nutritional Info

Calories 396

Carbs 41g

Fat 12g

Protein 38g

Vegetables with Pesto Sole

Serves: 2

Preparation Time: 20 minutes

Ingredients

Pesto (3 tablespoons)

Onion (1 ½ cups, chopped)

Asparagus (2 cups, cut up)

Vinegar (2 tablespoons)

Sole/flounder (8 oz.)

Black pepper

Mushrooms (2 cups, sliced)

Garlic (1 clove, crushed)

Fish stock (1 ½ cups)

Directions

1. Set oven to 350F and coat baking dish with cooking spray.
2. Heat skillet, coat with cooking spray and sauté garlic, asparagus, mushrooms and onions. Cook for 5 minutes then add broth and vinegar.
3. Transfer vegetable mixture to baking dish then add fish and coat with pesto. Bake for 15 minutes.
4. Serve.

Nutritional Info

Calories 377

Carbs 37g

Fat 11g

Protein 36g

Tuscan Pork

Serves: 1

Preparation Time: 25 minutes

Ingredients

Ground mustard (1/2 teaspoon)

Worcestershire sauce (1 teaspoon)

Olive oil (1 ½ teaspoons)

Onion (1/3 cup, sliced thin)

Tomato puree (1/4 cup)

Lemon juice (1 tablespoon, freshly squeezed)

Canned garbanzo beans (1/8 cup, slightly crushed)

Black pepper (1/8 teaspoon)

Herb dressing (1/2 cup)

Pork cutlets (3 oz.)

Mushrooms (1 cup, sliced)

Tomato (1/2, sliced)

Black pepper

Directions

1. Combine ¼ cup of dressing, Worcestershire sauce, pepper and mustard in a bowl.
2. Heat skillet and add ¾ teaspoon of oil; add water and dressing mixture. Put onions and cutlets into sauce and coat thoroughly.
3. Heat leftover in another skillet and sauté mushrooms and beans; cook for 5 minutes and add leftover dressing and puree.
4. Add vegetables to pork and mix together.
5. Serve pork with tomato slice. Top with black pepper and lemon juice.

Nutritional Info

Calories 344 Carbs 36g Fat 11g

Protein 27g

Pork Fillet and Fennel

Serves: 2

Preparation Time: 60 minutes

Ingredients

Pork tenderloin (7 oz.)

Olive oil (1 ¼ tablespoons)

Orange zest (2 teaspoons, grated)

Orange juice (1/4 cup, freshly squeezed)

Apples (2 cups, sliced)

Fennel (1 bulb, but in quarters)

White wine (1 tablespoon)

Capers (2 tablespoons)

Cinnamon (1 teaspoon)

Spinach (10 oz., steamed)

Directions

1. Set oven to 350F.
2. Slice pork and fennel into 4 parts equally. Heat oil in an oven proof skillet and cook pork and fennel until slightly golden.
3. Coat with wine and add zest. Cover pot and put into oven.
4. Bake for 30 minutes. Place apple slices onto a coated baking sheet and bake for 5 minutes.
5. Serve pork with spinach; place apples on the side with orange juice and capers.

Nutritional Info

Calories 354

Carbs 39g

Fat 12g

Protein 27g

Pork Medallion with Blueberries and Pears

Serves: 1

Preparation Time: 60 minutes

Ingredients

Olive oil (1 ¾ teaspoons)

Cider vinegar (1 tablespoon)

Pork tenderloin (3.5 oz., sliced)

Blueberries (1/2 cup)

Water (1 tablespoon)

Soy sauce (1/2 teaspoon)

Celery salt (1/8 teaspoon)

Scallion (1/2 cup, sliced)

Dijon mustard (2 teaspoons)

Brown sugar (1 teaspoon)

Pear (1/2, diced)

Mint (2 teaspoons, chopped)

Lemon juice (1 teaspoon, freshly squeezed)

Red wine vinegar (2 tablespoons)

Black pepper (1/8 teaspoon)

Romaine lettuce (4 cups, shredded)

Directions

1. Add mustard, brown sugar, 1 teaspoon oil and cider vinegar to a bowl; whisk together to combine and put pork into mixture.
2. Coat pork thoroughly and place in fridge for 30 minutes.
3. Heat a skillet and coat with cooking spray then add pork along with marinade to pot; cook for 15-20 minutes until pork is thoroughly cooked.
4. Add blueberries, water, lemon juice, pears and mint; cook for 5 minutes or until thoroughly heated.

5. Mix together leftover oil, red wine vinegar, black pepper, soy sauce and celery salt in a large bowl. Add lettuce and scallions to mixture and toss.
6. Serve pork with lettuce.

Nutritional Info

Calories 352

Carbs 29g

Fat 10g

Protein 27g

Apple Compote and Pork

Serves: 1

Preparation Time: 30 minutes

Ingredients

Olive oil (2 teaspoons)

Onion (1/2, sliced)

Applesauce (1/4 cup, unsweetened)

Celery salt (1/8 teaspoon)

Water (2 teaspoons)

Herbed lemon seasoning (1/4 teaspoon)

Vegetable broth (2 tablespoons)

Pork tenderloin (3.5 oz.)

Granny Smith (1, core removed and diced0

Cider vinegar (2 tablespoons)

Cinnamon (1/8 teaspoon)

Lemon juice (1 tablespoon, freshly squeezed)

Mushrooms (2 cups, sliced)

Directions

1. Heat a teaspoon of oil in a skillet. Cook pork for 10 minutes until slightly golden.
2. Add apple, vinegar, cinnamon, lemon juice, herb seasoning, onion, applesauce, celery salt and water to the skillet. Cook for 5 minutes.
3. Heat leftover oil in another skillet and sauté mushrooms for 5 minutes.
4. Serve pork with mushrooms.

Nutritional Info

Calories 338

Carbs 35g

Fat 12g

Protein 26g

Chicken Parmesan and Squash

Serves: 4

Preparation Time: 30 minutes

Ingredients

Chicken breasts (14 oz., skinless and boneless)

Garlic powder

Tomato and basil sauce (2 ½ cups)

Rosemary (dried)

Basil (dried)

Black pepper

Olive oil (1 tablespoon)

Vegan mozzarella (1/2 cup, shredded)

Oregano (dried)

Spaghetti squash (8 cups, cooked)

Directions

1. Set oven to 375F. Use garlic powder and black pepper to season chicken.
2. Heat oil in a skillet and cook chicken for 10 minutes or until thoroughly cooked.
3. Place chicken into a baking dish and add herbs, sauce and cheese. Bake for 10 minutes until cheese is golden.
4. Take chicken from sauce and place sauce into a microwavable dish along with squash. Stir to combine.
5. Serve squash with chicken.

Nutritional Info

Calories 359

Carbs 38g

Fat 10g

Protein 30g

Rosemary Chicken

Serves: 2

Preparation Time: 60 minutes

Ingredients

Garlic (1 clove, crushed)

Vegetable broth (1 cup)

Rosemary (3 teaspoons, fresh)

Chicken breast (6 oz., boneless and pounded)

White wine (1/4 cup)

Cauliflower (4 cups)

Olive oil (1 teaspoon)

Spinach (10 cups)

Butter (1 teaspoon)

Cornstarch (2 teaspoons)

Vegan mozzarella (1/4 cup)

Directions

1. Heat oil in a skillet and sauté garlic for 3 minutes until fragrant.
2. Add spinach, a teaspoon of rosemary and a ¼ of broth; cover pot and cook for 4 minutes until spinach is wilted.
3. In another skillet, melt butter and cook chicken for 10 minutes or until thoroughly cooked. Transfer chicken to pot with spinach.
4. Combine remaining broth with starch and add to chicken and spinach along with wine; cook until mixture is thick. Prepare cauliflower by steaming.
5. Top chicken with cheese and serve with cauliflower.

Nutritional Info

Calories 389 Carbs 38g

Fat 13g

Protein 31g

Seared Salmon, Spinach and Balsamic Syrup

Serves: 1

Preparation Time: 30 minutes

Ingredients

Balsamic vinegar (1/4 cup)

Spinach (5 cups)

Salmon filet (4 oz.)

Mandarin oranges (1/4 cup)

Honey (2 teaspoons)

Black pepper

Olive oil (1 teaspoon)

Directions

1. Add honey and vinegar to a small pot, whisk together and cook until mixture boils. Lower heat and cook for 7 minutes until syrup is formed.
2. Heat skillet and coat with cooking spray. Add spinach to skillet and cook for 3 minutes until wilted.
3. Use oil to coat salmon all over then place into a coated skillet with the skin side down. Cook for 5 minutes then flip fish and cook for 3 minutes. Test fish if thoroughly cooked.
4. Serve fish with spinach; drizzle with balsamic reduction.

Nutritional Info

Calories 334

Carbs 28g

Fat 12g

Protein 27g

Salmon and Asian Fruit Salsa

Serves: 1

Preparation Time: 45 minutes

Ingredients

Salmon steak (4 oz.)

Ginger (1 teaspoon, chopped)

Hot sauce

Blackberries (3/4 cup)

Green beans (1 ½ cups)

Soy sauce (2 teaspoons)

Dill (1/2 teaspoon)

Salsa (1/2 cup)

Blueberries (3/4 cup, slightly crushed)

Olive oil (1/2 teaspoon)

Directions

1. Coat baking dish with cooking spray and put salmon into dish.
2. Combine soy sauce, dill, hot sauce and ginger in a bowl and pour over salmon. Steam green beans.
3. Add fruit and salsa to a bowl and gently mix together, mashing a little bit.
4. Serve fish with salsa and beans.

Nutritional Info

Calories 343

Carbs 37g

Fat 10g

Protein 30g

Salsa Chicken

Serves: 1

Preparation Time: 60 minutes

Ingredients

Chicken breast (3 oz.)

Vegan mozzarella (1 ½ tablespoons)

Green beans (2 cups, steamed)

Salsa (1/2 cup)

Peach (1)

Guacamole (2 tablespoons)

Directions

1. Set oven to 350F.
2. Coat baking dish and place chicken into dish and top with salsa and cheese.
3. Bake for 20 minutes.
4. Serve with beans, peach and guacamole.

Nutritional Info

Calories 343

Carbs 41g

Fat 10g

Protein 29g

Braised Celery and Scallops

Serves: 1

Preparation Time: 20 minutes

Ingredients

Butter (1 ½ teaspoons)

Black pepper

Vegetable broth (1/2 cup, no salt)

Carrots (1, shredded)

Cardamom (1 teaspoon)

Olive oil (1 teaspoon)

Scallops (4.5 oz.)

Celery (2 stalks, diced)

Green apple (1, core removed, chopped)

Ginger (1/2 teaspoon, grated)

Walnuts (1 tablespoon, crushed)

Directions

1. Melt butter in a skillet and cook scallops for 8 minutes or until done.
2. Heat broth and braise celery until slightly cooked; add remaining vegetables, mix together and heat thoroughly.
3. Serve scallops with braised vegetable mix.

Nutritional Info

Calories 336

Carbs 37g

Fat 11g

Protein 24g

Seafood Pizza

Serves: 3

Preparation Time: 1 hour 30 minutes

Ingredients

Zucchini (2 cups, shredded)

Oat flour (1/4 cup)

Rosemary (2 teaspoons, dried)

Egg whites (4)

Vegan Parmesan (1/2 cup, grated)

Olive oil (2 ½ teaspoons)

For topping:

Basil (1 teaspoon)

Tomato paste (1 cup)

Mushrooms (4 cups, chopped)

Vegan mozzarella (1/3 cup)

Bell pepper (1, chopped)

Rosemary (1 teaspoon)

Tomato (1, chopped)

Cod (3 oz., chopped)

Onion (1 ½ cups, cut into rings)

Bell pepper (1, yellow, chopped)

Directions

1. Set oven at 400F.
2. Combine zucchini, flour, rosemary, egg whites, parmesan and olive oil in a bowl.
3. Coat pie dish with cooking spray and push dough into dish; bake for 40 minutes.

4. Take crust from oven and cool for 15 minutes and then put onto a baking tray.
5. Combine dried spices with tomato paste and spread onto crust.
6. Add toppings on to crust and bake for 20 minutes.
7. Cool and serve.

Nutritional Info

Calories 286

Carbs 27g

Fat 11g

Protein 23g

Curried Eggplant and Salmon

Serves: 1

Preparation Time: 30 minutes

Ingredients

Eggplant (1, sliced into rounds)

Olive oil (1 teaspoon)

Salmon (3.5 oz.)

Cherry tomatoes (15, cut into halves)

Curry (1 teaspoon)

Black pepper

Old Bay seasoning (1 teaspoon)

Directions

1. Set oven at 450°F.
2. Remove stem of eggplant and slice into round pieces. Use foil to line 2 baking trays and coat with cooking spray.
3. Coat eggplant with cooking spray then toss with black pepper and curry; place onto one of the lined trays. Use oil to coat fish and season with old bay seasoning.
4. Put both trays into oven. Bake eggplants for 3 minutes and remove from heat. Add tomatoes to tray and flip eggplant pieces and coat with cooking spray again. Return tray to oven and cook for an additional 3 minutes. Take salmon and vegetables from oven.
5. Serve.

Nutritional Info

Calories 368

Carbs 51g

Fat 8g

Protein 29g

Spanish Seafood Medley

Serves: 2

Preparation Time: 30 minutes

Ingredients

Olive oil (1 tablespoon)

Roasted red pepper (1/3 cup, chopped)

Sweet paprika (1 teaspoon)

Black pepper

White wine (1/4 cup, dry)

Tomatoes (1 cup, chopped)

Artichoke hearts (8 oz.)

Haddock (5 oz.)

Garlic (2 tablespoons)

Thyme (1 teaspoon)

Saffron (1/2 teaspoon)

Clam juice (1 ½ cups)

Bay leaf (1)

Green beans (2 cups)

Canned garbanzo (1/2 cup, drained)

Shrimp (2 oz., uncooked)

Directions

1. Heat oil in a deep skillet and sauté peppers and garlic for 1 minute. Add paprika, black pepper, thyme and saffron; mix together and cook for 2 minutes, stirring frequently.

2. Add clam juice, bay leaf, wine and cook for 1 minute until mixture comes to a boil. Add green beans, garbanzo beans, tomatoes, artichoke and cook for 3 minutes then lower flame.
3. Add haddock, try putting it under the vegetables and cover pot; cook for 2 minutes then flip haddock and put in shrimp.
4. Cook for an additional 5 minutes or until shrimp is pink and fish is flaky.
5. Serve.

Nutritional Info

Calories 390

Carbs 43g

Fat 10g

Protein 29g

Stuffed Peppers

Serves: 2

Preparation Time: 1 hour 20 minutes

Ingredients

Olive oil (1 ½ teaspoons)

Garlic (4 cloves, diced)

Canned kidney beans (1/4 cup)

Egg whites (4)

Curry powder (2 teaspoons, spicy)

Celery salt (1/8 teaspoon)

Chili powder (1/8 teaspoon)

Hot sauce (1/8 teaspoon)

Bell peppers (4)

Onion (1 cup, diced)

Mushrooms (1 cup, diced)

Bell pepper (1, red, diced)

Tofu (9 oz., firm)

Dry mustard (1/2 teaspoon)

Cinnamon (1/8 teaspoon)

Turmeric (1/8 teaspoon)

Directions

1. Set oven to 400F.
2. Heat oil in a skillet and add onion, mushrooms, red pepper, onion and kidney beans. Cook for 5-10 minutes until veggies are tender; take from heat and cool.
3. Transfer cooled veggies to a bowl with tofu, hot sauce, eggs and spices; mix together until thoroughly combined.

4. Remove stems from bell peppers and take out seeds inside. Remove a bit of skin from the bottom of peppers if necessary so that they don't tilt.
5. Coat baking dish and stuff peppers with tofu mixture and place into dish. Use foil to cover dish and bake for 60 minutes.
6. Serve warm.

Nutritional Info

Calories 387

Carbs 44g

Fat 13g

Protein 28g

Spaghetti with Cheesy Mushroom Sauce

Serves: 4

Preparation Time: 30 minutes

Ingredients

Spaghetti squash (6 lbs. or more)

Olive oil (3/4 cup)

Bell pepper (1/2 cup, chopped)

Mushrooms (8 oz., sliced)

Coconut milk (7 oz.)

Coconut cream (1 cup)

Oregano (1 teaspoon)

Vegan cheddar (3/4 cup, shredded)

Chicken breast (8 oz., ground)

Vegetable broth (1/2 cup, no salt)

Onions (1 ½ cups)

Canned tomatoes (14 oz., diced)

Basil (1 teaspoon)

Vegan Parmesan (4 teaspoons)

Directions

1. Pierce squash all over about 7 times and microwave for 6 minutes, turn over and microwave for an additional 6 minutes. You may also place squash in a coated baking dish and bake for 10 minutes. Take squash from oven and put aside to cool.
2. Heat a teaspoon of oil in a skillet and cook ground chicken for 5 minutes adding broth to avoid sticking. Take from heat and put aside until needed.
3. Heat leftover oil in another skillet and sauté mushrooms, onion and pepper; cook for 5 minutes until veggies are soft. Add coconut milk, basil, black pepper,

tomatoes, leftover broth and oregano; put in chicken and cook for 10 minutes. Stir in coconut cream and heat thoroughly until mixture has thickened.

4. Cut squash, take out seeds and use a fork to pull flesh of squash. Place onto dishes and top with chicken mixture.
5. Sprinkle with Parmesan and serve.

Nutritional Info

Calories 324

Carbs 34g

Fat 12g

Protein 28g

Stuffed Zucchini

Serves: 2

Preparation Time: 30 minutes

Ingredients

Onion (1 cup, sliced thin)

Caraway seeds (2 teaspoons)

Italian chicken sausage (2 links)

Summer squash (2 cups, sliced in half)

Vegetable broth (1 cup, unsalted)

Hot sauce (1 teaspoon)

Parsley (1/4 cup, chopped)

Zucchini (3 cups, sliced in halves)

Tomatoes (3 cups, diced)

Vegan mozzarella (1/3 cup, shredded)

Directions

1. Set oven to 375℉.
2. Heat a skillet and add 2 tablespoons of broth, hot sauce, parsley, sausage, onion and caraway seeds. Cook for 5 minutes or until sausage is golden all over; remove from heat and put aside until needed.
3. Place ½ of squash and zucchini into a baking dish and fill with sausage mixture; repeat with leftover squash and zucchini.
4. Add leftover broth, cover with foil and bake for 20 minutes. Remove foil, top with cheese and bake for an additional 10 minutes.
5. Serve.

Nutritional Info

Calories 345 Carbs 39g

Fat 11g

Protein 28g

Sweet and Sour Shrimp

Serves: 2

Preparation Time: 30 minutes

Ingredients

Olive oil (1 teaspoon)

Grapefruits (2)

Steel cut oats (1/3 cup, cooked)

Cherry tomatoes (3/4 cup, cut into halves)

Black pepper

Shrimp (7 oz.)

Zucchini (2 cups, sliced in thin strips)

Apple (1 cup, chopped)

Olive oil (2 teaspoon)

Directions

1. Heat half of oil in a skillet and sauté shrimp for 5 minutes then squeeze half of a grapefruit over shrimp and cook until liquid evaporates. Take shrimp from pot and put aside.
2. Add leftover oil along with zucchini and black pepper. Cook until tender then add oats.
3. Peel the remaining whole grapefruit and slice. Squeeze the half of grapefruit into a bowl along with oil and black pepper.
4. Serve oats with zucchini, shrimp and grapefruit. Add grapefruit mixture and toss.

Nutritional Info

Calories 334

Carbs 39g

Fat 10g

Protein 25g

Teriyaki Halibut

Serves: 2

Preparation Time: 40 minutes

Ingredients

Olive oil (3 teaspoons)

Teriyaki (1/4 cup, preferably low carb)

Leeks (2, diced)

Herbed lemon seasoning (4 teaspoons)

Mandarin (1/2 cup)

Cauliflower (2 cups)

Halibut (7 oz., filet)

Bok choy (1 ½ cups, chopped)

Garlic (1 teaspoon, diced)

Nutmeg (1/2 teaspoon)

Baby spinach (4 cups)

Vinegar (1 tablespoon)

Directions

1. Set oven to 325°F.
2. Coat baking dish with 1 teaspoon of oil. Put in halibut, teriyaki sauce and cover dish with foil; bake for 30 minutes.
3. Heat leftover oil in a skillet, add leeks, seasoning, bok choy, cauliflower and garlic; cook for 5-8 minutes.
4. Serve vegetables with halibut along with spinach and mandarin. Drizzle spinach with vinegar.

Nutritional Info

Calories 369 Carbs 40g Fat 11g

Protein 33g

Tofu Marinara

Serves: 4

Preparation Time: 30 minutes

Ingredients

Tofu (24 oz., firm)

Canned black beans (1 ½ cup, drained)

Onion (1 cup, diced)

Bell peppers (6, cut into strips)

Olive oil (4 teaspoons)

Tomato sauce (1 cup)

Zucchini (6 cups, chopped)

Vegan mozzarella (1 cup, shredded)

Herb seasoning (Mrs. Dash)

Directions

1. Cut tofu into cubes.
2. Heat oil in a skillet and cook tofu until golden then add beans and tomato sauce.
3. Add vegetables and seasoning; stir gently and heat thoroughly until vegetables are softened.
4. Top with cheese and cook until it melts.
5. Serve.

Nutritional Info

Calories 341

Carbs 40g

Fat 11g

Protein 26g

Baked Cabbage and Meatballs

Serves: 3

Preparation Time: 2 hours 30 minutes

Ingredients

Cabbage (8 cups, cut into large sections)

Tomato sauce (8 oz.)

Water (1 ½ cups)

Ground beef (11 oz.)

Olive oil (1 tablespoon)

Blueberries (1 cup, slightly mashed)

Canned tomatoes (16 oz., diced)

Honey (1 teaspoon)

Vinegar (2 tablespoons)

Onion (1 cup, diced)

Lemon juice (2 tablespoons, freshly squeezed)

Peaches (1 cup, slightly mashed)

Egg whites (2)

Directions

1. Set oven to 325F.
2. Coat roasting pan with cooking spray and add cabbage to pan.
3. Add tomato sauce, vinegar, lemon juice, tomatoes and water to a saucepan; cook until thoroughly heated then take from heat.
4. Put meat, oil, egg and meat into a bowl and use hands to combine and for into meatballs. Add meatballs to roasting pan along with tomato sauce. Cover with foil and bake for 2 hours.
5. Serve warm with mashed berries and peaches on the side.

Nutritional Info

Calories 344 Carbs 39g Fat 11g

Protein 28g

Check out other Amazon best sellers from the Recipe Junkie family! Join our FREE newsletter!

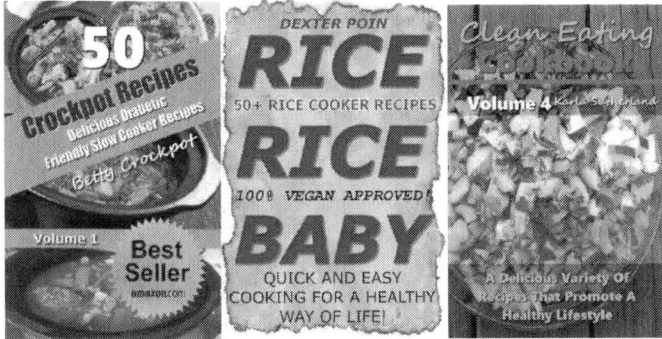

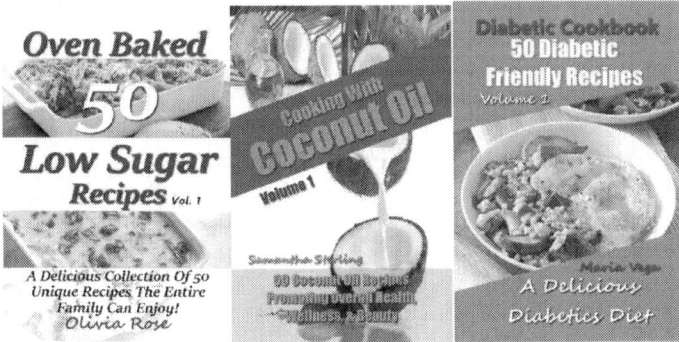

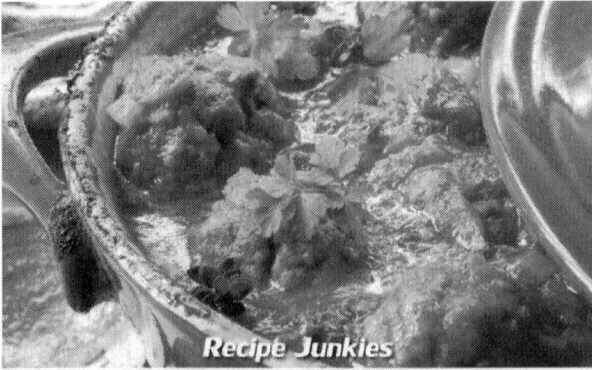

Recipe Junkies

CROCKPOT
R E C I P E S

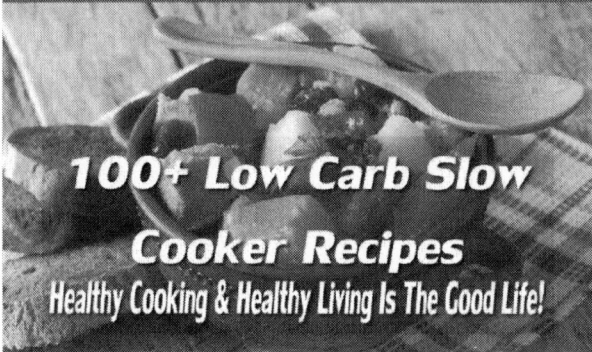

100+ Low Carb Slow Cooker Recipes
Healthy Cooking & Healthy Living Is The Good Life!

The information provided in this book is designed to provide helpful information on the subjects discussed. This book is not meant to be used, nor should it be used, to diagnose or treat any medical condition. For diagnosis or treatment of any medical problem, consult your own physician. The publisher and author are not responsible for any specific health or allergy needs that may require medical supervision and are not liable for any damages or negative consequences from any treatment, action, application or preparation, to any person reading or following the information in this book. References are provided for informational purposes only and do not constitute endorsement of any websites or other sources. Readers should be aware that the websites listed in this book may change.

These recipes are not intended to be any type of Medical advice. ALL individuals must consult their Doctors first and should always receive their meal plans from a qualified practitioner. . These recipes are not intended to heal, or cure anyone from any kind of illness, or disease.

Printed in Great Britain
by Amazon